AF700206

Advances in Industrial Control

Springer
London
Berlin
Heidelberg
New York
Barcelona
Hong Kong
Milan
Paris
Santa Clara
Singapore
Tokyo

Other titles published in this Series:

H_∞ Aerospace Control Design: A VSTOL Flight Application
R.A. Hyde

Neural Network Engineering in Dynamic Control Systems
Edited by Kenneth Hunt, George Irwin and Kevin Warwick

Neuro-Control and its Applications
Sigeru Omatu, Marzuki Khalid and Rubiyah Yusof

Energy Efficient Train Control
P.G. Howlett and P.J. Pudney

Hierarchical Power Systems Control: Its Value in a Changing Industry
Marija D. Ilic and Shell Liu

System Identification and Robust Control
Steen Tøffner-Clausen

Genetic Algorithms for Control and Signal Processing
K.F. Man, K.S. Tang, S. Kwong and W.A. Halang

Advanced Control of Solar Plants
E.F. Camacho, M. Berenguel and F.R. Rubio

Control of Modern Integrated Power Systems
E. Mariani and S.S. Murthy

Advanced Load Dispatch for Power Systems: Principles, Practices and Economies
E. Mariani and S.S. Murthy

Supervision and Control for Industrial Processes
Björn Sohlberg

Modelling and Simulation of Human Behaviour in System Control
Pietro Carlo Cacciabue

Modelling and Identification in Robotics
Krzysztof Kozlowski

Spacecraft Navigation and Guidance
Maxwell Noton

Robust Estimation and Failure Detection
Rami Mangoubi

Adaptive Internal Model Control
Aniruddha Datta

Price-Based Commitment Decisions in the Electricity Market
Eric Allen and Marija Ilić

Compressor Surge and Rotating Stall: Modeling and Control
Jan Tommy Gravdahl and Olav Egeland

Olivier Haas

Radiotherapy Treatment Planning

New System Approaches

With 138 Figures

Springer

Olivier Cyrille Louis Haas, PhD, MSc, BEng, DUT
Control Theory and Applications Centre, Coventry University, Priory Street, Coventry CV1 5FB, UK

ISBN 978-1-4471-1210-5

British Library Cataloguing in Publication Data
Haas, Olivier C.L.
Radiotherapy treatment planning : new system approaches. - (Advances in industrial control)
1. Radiotherapy - Planning
I. Title
615.8'42
ISBN 978-1-4471-1210-5 ISBN 978-1-4471-0821-4 (eBook)
DOI 10.1007/978-1-4471-0821-4
Library of Congress Cataloging-in-Publication Data
Haas, Olivier C.L. (Olivier Cyrille Louis)
Radiotherapy treatment planning : new system approaches / Olivier C.L. Haas.
p. cm. -- (Advances in industrial control)
Includes bibliographical references.
ISBN 978-1-4471-1210-5
1. Cancer--Radiotherapy--Planning. 2. Cancer--Radiotherapy--Data processing. I. Title. II. Series.
[DNLM: 1. Radiotherapy Planning, Computer-Assisted.
2. Radiotherapy Dosage. WN 250.5.R2 H112r 1998]
RC271.R3H38 1998
616.99'40642--dc21
DNLM/DLC 98-33473
for Library of Congress CIP

Apart from any fair dealing for the purposes of research or private study, or criticism or review, as permitted under the Copyright, Designs and Patents Act 1988, this publication may only be reproduced, stored or transmitted, in any form or by any means, with the prior permission in writing of the publishers, or in the case of reprographic reproduction in accordance with the terms of licences issued by the Copyright Licensing Agency. Enquiries concerning reproduction outside those terms should be sent to the publishers.

© Springer-Verlag London Limited 1999
Softcover reprint of the hardcover 1st edition 1999

The use of registered names, trademarks, etc. in this publication does not imply, even in the absence of a specific statement, that such names are exempt from the relevant laws and regulations and therefore free for general use.

The publisher makes no representation, express or implied, with regard to the accuracy of the information contained in this book and cannot accept any legal responsibility or liability for any errors or omissions that may be made.

Typesetting: Camera ready by author

69/3830-543210 Printed on acid-free paper

Advances in Industrial Control

Series Editors

Professor Michael J. Grimble, Professor of Industrial Systems and Director
Professor Michael A. Johnson, Professor of Control Systems and Deputy Director

Industrial Control Centre
Department of Electronic and Electrical Engineering
University of Strathclyde
Graham Hills Building
50 George Street
Glasgow G1 1QE
United Kingdom

Series Advisory Board

Professor Dr-Ing J. Ackermann
DLR Institut für Robotik und Systemdynamik
Postfach 1116
D82230 Weßling
Germany

Professor I.D. Landau
Laboratoire d'Automatique de Grenoble
ENSIEG, BP 46
38402 Saint Martin d'Heres
France

Dr D.C. McFarlane
Department of Engineering
University of Cambridge
Cambridge CB2 1QJ
United Kingdom

Professor B. Wittenmark
Department of Automatic Control
Lund Institute of Technology
PO Box 118
S-221 00 Lund
Sweden

Professor D.W. Clarke
Department of Engineering Science
University of Oxford
Parks Road
Oxford OX1 3PJ
United Kingdom

Professor Dr -Ing M. Thoma
Westermannweg 7
D-30419 Hannover
Germany

Professor H. Kimura
Department of Mathematical Engineering and Information Physics
Faculty of Engineering
The University of Tokyo
7-3-1 Hongo
Bunkyo Ku
Tokyo 113
Japan

Professor A.J. Laub
College of Engineering - Dean's Office
University of California
One Shields Avenue
Davis
California 95616-5294
United States of America

Professor J.B. Moore
Department of Systems Engineering
The Australian National University
Research School of Physical Sciences
GPO Box 4
Canberra
ACT 2601
Australia

Dr M.K. Masten
Texas Instruments
2309 Northcrest
Plano
TX 75075
United States of America

Professor Ton Backx
AspenTech Europe B.V.
De Waal 32
NL-5684 PH Best
The Netherlands

Science sans conscience n'est que ruine de l'âme.

François Rabelais (1494-1553)

SERIES EDITORS' FOREWORD

The series *Advances in Industrial Control* aims to report and encourage technology transfer in control engineering. The rapid development of control technology impacts all areas of the control discipline. New theory, new controllers, actuators, sensors, new industrial processes, computer methods, new applications, new philosophies, ..., new challenges. Much of this development work resides in industrial reports, feasibility study papers and the reports of advanced collaborative projects. The series offers an opportunity for researchers to present an extended exposition of such new work in all aspects of industrial control for wider and rapid dissemination.

This monograph reports multi-disciplinary research comprising the areas of medicine, control engineering and computer systems. Radiotherapy treatment is distressing at the best of times so work which seeks to enhance the accuracy of the process and improve the planning of patient treatment is to be highly commended. Olivier Haas, the author of this monograph, has modelled the radiotherapy delivery process and used optimization theory to solve radiotherapy treatment planning problems. The resulting work has also progressed to successful practical experiments and indeed the research is continuing to generate new results.

The application of control engineering in medical science is a fairly new and growing area. This monograph is the first medical-control engineering entry to the Advances in Industrial Control series. It is to be hoped that it is not the last but first in a growing collection of bio-medical applications volumes.

M.J. Grimble and M.A. Johnson
Industrial Control Centre
Glasgow, Scotland, UK

PREFACE

The idea of reporting my research work within this monograph came to light during the oral examination of my PhD thesis on 'Optimisation and Control Systems Modelling in Radiotherapy Treatment Planning'. This original research work which culminated in 1996 by a series of experiments carried out at Walsgrave Hospital NHS Trust, Coventry in collaboration with Leicester Royal Infirmary, Leicester. It formed the basis for the establishment of a new Biomedical Control Research Group within the Control Theory and Applications Centre, Coventry University.

The overall aim of the collaborative Research with Walsgrave Hospital was to design an intelligent oncology workstation, which could automatically outline regions of interest, inhomogeneous structures and cancerous regions prior to optimising the resulting treatment plan. This overall research programme is now becoming a practical reality. Semi automatic organ segmentation software has now been developed whose output can be used by the optimisation software currently being refined. The latter refinements take into account practical aspects linked to the actual delivery of radiotherapy treatments using beam intensity modulation, e.g. limitations of the beam modulation apparatus and influence of patient movement.

A unique aspect of the intensity modulated radiation therapy problem dealt with in this monograph is the multidisciplinary nature of the work which required effective collaboration between engineers, scientists and clinicians.

It should be equally interesting for control engineers, computer scientists and medical physicists. Medical physicists should find an interesting summary of current techniques used to solve the optimisation problems in radiotherapy treatment planning. Computer scientists may be interested by the application and customisation of multi-objective genetic algorithms to solve radiotherapy treatment planning optimisation problems. Control engineers should find this book enlightening as it demonstrates that control engineering is not only limited to traditional industrial processes but can also be applied to solve problems related to physics and medicine. It should be particularly interesting for MSc and PhD students in the field of medical physics and biomedical engineering.

The most interesting aspect of the monograph is that it reports the use of novel approaches based both on deterministic (i.e. model based) and heuristic or guided random search (i.e. model independent) techniques to solve a wide range of problems facing physicists and treatment planners in the area of radiotherapy physics. In particular, the beam orientation problem, the optimisation of the optimal combination of beam weight and wedge angle, and the optimisation of beam intensity modulation are all dealt with in this work. This should prove invaluable for anyone involved in subsequent studies concerning the problems dealt with in this single volume.

The research work reported includes novel theoretical results which are demonstrated practically using the latest measurement techniques in the field of radiation dosimetry.

Systems modelling techniques have been used to model the effect of intensity modulated X-ray beams. The model proved to be adequate in replicating intensity modulated dose distributions in water.

Adopting a model based approach, the optimisation of beam intensity modulation is performed using a weighted iterative least squares (ILS) technique modified to allow an adaptive scaling of the error to improve the performance of the general least squares algorithm. The influence of various modifications of the information matrix is also studied and it is concluded that some of the schemes proposed are superior to ILS with a fixed information matrix. Cautious least squares techniques have also been investigated to apply constraints on the beam weightings. This is another novel approach to the optimisation of beam intensity modulation.

Multi-objective genetic algorithms (MOGAs) have been used to optimise beam weights and wedge angles as well as coplanar beam orientation. Again this is a novel application which makes use of a specialised MOGA to solve optimisation problems that have been previously solved with simulated annealing or traditional genetic algorithms.

The overall approach is demonstrated practically using both traditional measurement techniques such as film and more modern techniques such as gel dosimeter. A brief description of the characteristics of each dosimeter is given, which is particularly interesting in the case of the gel dosimeter, as such a technique is still very much in its infancy.

Finally it gives me great pleasure to acknowledge the people who have made this monograph possible. In particular, I would like to thank Dr John Mills, Radiotherapy Physics Manager at Walsgrave Hospital NHS Trust, Coventry, for his help in the area of radiotherapy physics and his continuing enthusiasm. I am particularly grateful to his commitment to the project and his help with respect to the experimental work which was carried out outside normal working hours.

I would also like to thank Dr M. R. Katebi for suggesting the idea of this monograph, Prof. M. J. Grimble and Prof. M. A. Johnson, editors of the monograph Series 'Advances in Industrial Control' for their comments and encouragement in pursuing this project.

Last but not least I would like to thank Dr K. J. Burnham, co-director of the Control Theory and Applications Centre, Coventry University, for his guidance and supervision throughout my PhD research programme and his help with the writing up of my PhD thesis and the polishing of this monograph.

Coventry, August, 1998 Olivier C L Haas

CONTENTS

NOMENCLATURE

The following lists the key terms and abbreviations that are used throughout the work.

BEV: Beam's eye view, i.e. patient as seen from the beam source, where the observer is looking at the patient along the beam path.

BTV: Biological target volume, volume of tissues including the tumour volume (GTV) and regions known to have, or considered to be at risk for containing microscopic extension of disease including regional lymph nodes.

CAX: Central axis.

Conformal radiotherapy: Radiotherapy technique which is able to deliver a high dose of radiation to the diseased tissues whilst at the same time ensuring that the dose delivered to healthy tissues is acceptable. It can be delivered both by shaping the beam so that they replicate the shape of the diseased regions as seen from the beam and by modulating the beam in field intensity.

CT: Computed tomography.

CTA/CTV: Clinical target area/volume, this is an anatomical-clinical concept.

d_{max}: Maximal dose measured from a single X-ray photon beam, usually normalised to 100%

DSAR Differential scatter air ratio.

EA: Evolutionary algorithm.

EC: Evolutionary computing.

ES: Evolution strategies.

FS: Field size defined in terms of length and width of a usually square or rectangular field. It is distance between two pairs of points located on the geometrical edge of the field that receive 50% of the dose received by the central axis at the point of equilibrium. This value has been used since 1978 to define field size by the British Institute of Radiology.

FSA: Fast simulated annealing.

GA: Genetic algorithm.

GTA/GTV: Gross tumour area/volume, this is the palpable or visible/demonstrable extent and location of the malignant growth.

HS: Hot spots, i.e. regions which receive a dose larger than 100% of the dose specified to the target.

IAP: In-air-profile, i.e. beam profile measured in the air. The IAP arises due to the use of a built-in flattening filter in the head of the linear accelerator that reduces the power of the beam at the centre of the field compared with the elemental beam power on the edge of the beam.

ILS: Iterative least squares.

IMRT: Intensity modulated radiation therapy, treatment technique which modulate the beam intensity via compensators of multileaf collimator apparatus to conform radiotherapy treatments to demanding prescriptions

Linac: Linear accelerator.

MLC: Multi-leaf collimator.

MOGA: Multi-objective genetic algorithm.

MOP: Multi-objective optimisation problem.

MRI: Magnetic resonance imaging.

NTCP: Normal tissue complication probability.

OARs: Organs at risk, these are normal tissues whose radiation sensitivity may significantly influence treatment planning and /or prescribed dose.

OHT: Other healthy tissue.

PTA/PTV: Prescribed target area/volume, this is a geometrical concept defined to select appropriate beam size and beam arrangements, taking into consideration the net effect of all possible geometrical variations and inaccuracies in order to ensure that the prescribed dose is actually absorbed by the CTV.

PSC: Patient specific compensators.

RBO: Region of beam overlap.

ROI: Regions of interest, includes PTA, OARs and all other body structures that are of importance when planning a radiotherapy treatment.

RTP: Radiotherapy treatment planning.

SA: Simulated annealing.

SAR: Scatter air ratio.

SSD: Source to skin distance.

TAR: Tissue air ratio.

TCP: Tumour control probability.

x_{max}: Depth at which equilibrium occurs, this is the depth at which the dose is maximal $d_{max} = 100\%$.

CHAPTER 1
INTRODUCTION AND BRIEF REVIEW OF DEVELOPMENTS IN RADIOTHERAPY

1.1 Introduction

Advances in computer technology in recent years have made a significant impact on all aspects of human life and this has raised expectations of successive generations in today's modern progressive world. Remarkable technological advances have been made in engineering and science, with the computer playing an increasingly important role in society at large. The medical profession has not escaped this revolution, with the emergence in recent years of techniques and technologies which doubtless could never have been considered a reality only a few decades ago.

Radiotherapy, which makes use of radiation to treat cancer, has steadily grown from the begining of the century, where treatment techniques and apparatus were very much experimental, to the present day, where most regional based hospitals offer radiotherapy as a standard form of patient care. The growing number of patients suffering from cancer and requiring radiotherapy treatment has prompted the need for increasingly efficient, repeatable and accurate means for ensuring that appropriate treatment is administered. Consequently, the drive to improve radiotherapy treatment, in order to enhance patient care, coupled with important issues concerning quality of life, should remain high on the biomedical-engineering research agenda. Indeed, it is against this background that the outcomes of the programme of research first presented in [1] are based. This work was carried out in collaboration with the Department of Clinical Physics and Bioengineering, Walsgrave Hospital NHS Trust, Coventry, in association with the Leicester Royal Infirmary, Leicester, the Queen Elizabeth Hospital, Birmingham and the Western General Hospital, Edinburgh.

The procedures involved in the delivery of radiotherapy treatment are such that it is now technically possible to deliver highly complex treatments that should reduce the risks of complication by minimising the dose delivered to healthy tissues and consequently improve the patients well being. The complexity of these new treatment techniques known as conformal radiotherapy or intensity modulated radiation therapy (IMRT) is such that there is a need to automate the treatment procedures both at the planning and at the delivery stage.

Optimisation algorithms can be used to assist clinicians to devise appropriate treatment plans for each patient. The selection of an appropriate radiotherapy treatment plan (RTP) involves many factors including patient physio-demographic data, age and health profile, type and anatomical location of cancer as well as the risk of complication. An excellent review of the subject can be found in [2, 3, 4], with an account of recent advances and associated technology being given in [3]. In this work attention is focused on optimising both traditional means of delivering radiotherapy and more modern IMRT techniques which modulate the radiation intensity across the beams.

Traditional radiotherapy treatment techniques have only limited means to modulate the beam intensity. This prompted clinicians and medical physicists to adopt a conservative approach by irradiating 'boxed' volumes which, in some cases, may be larger than strictly necessary to ensure total eradication of the cancer. IMRT, which has been seen as a refinement to traditional radiation therapy, offers the possibility to conform to complex prescriptions with a higher degree of accuracy [5, 6, 7, 8]. In particular, IMRT can shape and modulate the beams such that a high prescribed dose can be delivered to concave target volumes whilst at the same time sparing other healthy tissues. This results in an increased sparing of vital organs when compared to traditional radiotherapy which cannot conform to concave target volumes. This increased sparing of healthy tissues enables an escalation of dose delivered to the target [3]. By increasing the amount of radiation delivered to the cancerous region, whilst keeping the dose elsewhere low, improvements in the quality of treatment should hopefully lead, in turn, to improvements in the quality of life for patients receiving such treatment.

The work has been motivated largely through the ongoing need to develop an automated (or semi-automated) RTP system which could usefully exploit the widespread availability of modern computing hardware/software technology. Optimisation approaches have been developed and applied to a number of interrelated problems that are relevant to qualitative and quantitative improvements in RTP.

The approach followed in this work differs from that of previous researchers in the field in that the problem is formulated within the context of a control engineering framework. Techniques which are analogous to control theoretical design methodologies, used in the design of controllers for industrial plant, are employed here to obtain optimum values, in some sense, for the intensity modulated beams (IMBs). In particular, following a systems modelling and control approach a new two-dimensional matrix beam model which characterises the behaviour of a photon beam is developed. The route, from the initial concept stage to the fully refined model tested in a practical clinical environment is divided into Chap. 2 and 3. The background and preliminary modelling considerations are presented in Chap. 2 where mathematical expressions for the primary, the scatter, the penumbra, the in-air-profile, as well as patient contour correction and inhomogeneity correction are deduced from experimental measurements.

The mathematical abstraction that is necessary when developing the matrix based beam model, is dealt with mainly in Chap. 3. The beam model is built around the concept of separating the effect of radiation into primary and scatter components. A parallel beam is initially formulated in order to allow the design of optimisation methods to solve the so-called inverse problem of RTP. The model is then refined and a more realistic divergent pencil beam model is developed; this being inspired mainly from the point of view of developing a forward solving methodology. Both the parallel and divergent beam models are demonstrated and compared to measured data obtained from experimental trials undertaken at Walsgrave Hospital NHS Trust, Coventry. The appropriateness of the models in terms of their ability to replicate observed phenomena provided the necessary confidence to continue with the approach, to further refine and develop model based routines for optimising the IMBs.

In this work, the investigation into optimisation of the beams is pursued in two fundamentally different ways. The first, which is presented in Chap. 4, is to make use of an iterative least squares (ILS) procedure [9] which is tailored to the RTP problem. An extension of the approach is made by introducing a cautious least squares estimation scheme when constraints on the beam weight intensities and their discrete difference, or gradients, are imposed from physical considerations. The latter is used to determine a set of beam weights and wedge angles by solving a 'constrained inverse problem' [1]. It is shown that a modification of the information matrix, employing techniques that are similar to the use of forgetting factors and Kalman filtering in dynamic situations, can improve the overall performance in terms of convergence behaviour of the algorithm.

In Chap. 5, a forward solving methodology which makes use of a genetic algorithm (GA) approach [10] is presented. It is shown that GAs lend themselves well to the RTP problem, not only for solving the IMBs, but also for optimising the number and orientation of the beams as well as the combination of beam weights and wedge angles. In particular, a novel geometrical approach to solving the beam orientation problem is proposed which makes use of hybrid GAs including problem specific operators. It is also shown that the use of GAs provide a possible framework for utilising non quadratic cost functions, thus allowing increased flexibility, as well as the ability to handle multi-objective criteria, leading to the concept of a Pareto optimal solution set [11]. It is demonstrated that a multi-objective genetic algorithm (MOGA) implemented around the concept of Pareto optimality exhibits an increased degree of flexibility compared to the traditional weighted sum approach used in conventional RTP [1]. Both the ILS and GA approaches are found to work well using the developed parallel and divergent beam models, respectively. Clinical aspects, such as hot spot minimisation and the influence of combinations of different beam energies, have also been addressed.

The culmination of the work lies in a proposal for a suite of optimisation methodologies for solving problems encountered in RTP. In particular a novel hybrid approach to the solution of the IMB optimisation problem is proposed in Chap. 6. The hybrid approach combines both the inverse solution and the forwar solution based methodologies. Essentially the method of ILS is used first in conjunction with a parallel pencil beam in order to obtain an initial family of potential solutions and then a MOGA is used in conjunction with a divergent pencil beam model to widen the search space and seek alternative solutions. This yields a Pareto optimal set from which equitable solutions, in terms of a user defined performance index, may be selected.

The effect of the compensators is modelled such that compensator profiles can be deduced for optimised IMB profiles. Tool path generation code for a computer numerically controlled machined is then deduced to enable the manufacture of the patient specific compensators. Chapter 6 also presents the results of practical field trials in which a five field conformal treatment plan is tested on two semi-anatomical torso phantoms incorporating radiosensitive film and gel dosimeter. These tests provided valuable information with the results of the experimental field trials conducted at Walsgrave Hospital, NHS Trust, Coventry, in association with the Leicester Royal Infirmary, Leicester, being in good agreement with theoretical predictions. The overall results obtained from the trials serve to highlight the effectiveness of the developed approach as well as the ability of gel dosimeter to assess IMRT. The outcome was considered to be very encouraging and constituted the first attempt in the UK to actually realise beam intensity modulation practically.

Finally overall conclusions and suggestions for further work are presented in Chap. 7.

1.2 Historical Review of Developments in Radiotherapy

Before embarking on the study into improving radiotherapy treatment one cannot overlook the significant contributions of distinguished individuals in the field. As such a brief historical note is included. An excellent review of the historical development of X-rays and radioactivity in medicine can be found in the authoritative text by Richard F. Mould [12]. Other interesting reports on the early developments may be found in the review papers [2, 13].

In 1995, the first 100 years of radiology was celebrated in Birmingham, UK, [14], and 1996 marked the 100th anniversary of the first documented clinical radiation treatment performed by Leopold Freund in Vienna [12]. Since these early days radiotherapy has evolved from an experimental technique [13, 14] to a widely used treatment procedure for the eradication of cancer [2, 3, 15]. This has been made possible by a better understanding of the effect of radiation on human tissues [2, 3] and the developments of procedures to improve the selectivity of treatments [3, 5, 7, 9, 16, 17].

1.2.1 The Early Workers

The 19th century ended with some significant discoveries for the diagnostics and treatment of cancer. In 1895 Wilhelm Conrad Röntgen discovered X-rays in his laboratory at the Physical Institute of the Julius-Maximilian University of Würzburg in Bavaria. Radioactivity was discovered in 1896 by Antoine Henri Becquerel, and Marie Curie established that radium was a radioactive substance that could produce rays with an identical effect as X-rays, which became known as gamma-rays (γ-rays) [1, 12, 13].

The ability of X-rays to differentiate matter through their densities made it similarly attractive for clinicians and engineers. However, the relative carelessness in the handling of radiation in the early years led a large number of individuals, to suffer from radiation exposure. It was the observations of these secondary effects of radiation exposure, such as the loss of hair, that led to the early therapeutical use of radiation. Other early reported work included experiments with X and γ-rays to treat cancer and ulcers of various types [1, 12, 13]. These early treatments involved direct application of the radioactive substances to the superficial lesions. It is unfortunate to note that a large number of these early workers paid with their lives to achieve the remarkable advances made in the field; this being due largely to a lack of awareness of the dangers of radiation, and the need for adequate radiation protection equipment combined with the treatment procedures at that time.

1.2.2 Effect of Radiation on Human Tissues

Nowadays it is well known that, although X-rays can destroy cancerous cells and sterilise malignant tumours to cure cancer patients, they can also damage any normal tissue through which they traverse [3, 12]. It has also become apparent that the effects of radiation are progressive and may take weeks or even months to be noticed. This is due to the fact that cells condemned by radiation do not die instantly and may even reproduce themselves before being eliminated from the organism [2, 18].

This progressive alteration of cells has been found to be of advantage, allowing for the reduction in the risks of complication due to an over-dosage of healthy tissues. The radiation treatment is delivered in a number of fractions over a period of weeks, which allows normal tissues to regenerate themselves while the treatment of the cancer tissues accumulates. The increased ability of healthy cells to regenerate themselves compared to cancerous cells enables the clinicians to plan treatment so that cancerous cells are destroyed whilst only a minimum number of healthy cells are permanently affected.

Although originally introduced as early as 1919 [12, 13], dose fractionation in the delivery of radiotherapy treatment is still today an area of active research [19, 20, 21, 22]. Modern refinements combine dose fractionation with the use of substances that increase the relative sensitivity of cancerous cells by making them less resistant to radiation [23]; thus improving the so called 'differential effect' [24].

1.2.3 Improving the Physical Selectivity of Treatments

The term 'physical selectivity' of X-rays is defined as the dose delivered to the tumour relative to that delivered to normal tissues [24]. The earliest method used to increase, or improve, the physical selectivity was to use several beams from different directions so that they were superposed over the target. In this way, the dose received by the target is the sum of the doses from each beam within the target region [2, 12].

In the early days of radiotherapy, the lack of sufficient penetration of X-ray beams prevented their use for the so called 'deep seated' tumours, such as for example prostate cancer. As previously mentioned, the first successful treatment involved only skin cancer and other superficial lesions [1, 12, 13]. In addition, physicists often had to stop treatment due to more or less acute skin reaction. This was due to the fact that the skin irradiated by the treatment machines of the time received higher dose than the other tissues in the beam path. The development of megavoltage beams enabled the reduction of relative dose received by the skin, (the so called 'skin sparing effect') whilst at the same time increasing the penetration of the beam due to the process of physical interaction between X-ray photons and matter (see Chap. 2 and 3); the higher beam energies being less attenuated. Figure 1.1 shows various levels of central axis (CAX) percentage depth dose (%DD), indicating the penetration and skin sparing effect for different beam voltages; it is compiled from the Supplement 17 of the British Journal of Radiology [25]. Note that a revised version of the Supplement 17 on CAX %DD has recently been published in the Supplement 25 of the British Journal of Radiology [26].

It is now acknowledged that to improve the physical selectivity of X-rays it is required to determine the optimum number [27, 28] and orientation [2, 3, 7, 29, 30] of the beams involved. It is also necessary to optimise the beam shapes in order to accurately reproduce the 'beam's eye view' of the tumour [1, 2, 3] i.e. the shape of the target as viewed from the beam source. This can be achieved by making use of multi-leaf collimators (MLCs) in a static manner [3, 31, 32, 33, 34, 35] or other beam shaping devices [3, 32] whilst, at the same time, selecting the optimum intensity modulation devices, such as standard wedges [36, 37], patient specific compensators [38, 39, 40, 41, 42, 43] or dynamic MLCs in which the leaves are required to move during the treatment delivery [44, 45, 46, 47, 48, 49, 50].

All the above techniques, are aimed at improving the physical selectivity of radiotherapy treatment, and endeavour to ensure that a sufficient amount of radiation can be delivered to the diseased tissues while minimising that to normal tissues.

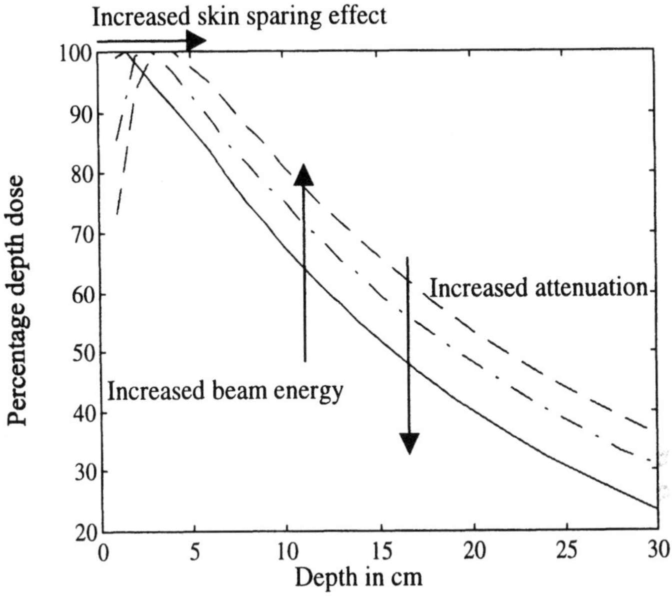

Fig. 1.1 Comparison between central axis percentage depth dose for three different beam energies (compiled from the Supplement 17 of the British Journal of Radiology): 6 MV, represented by solid line, 10 MV by dot-dashed line and 25 MV by dashed line

1.2.4 Development of Megavoltage X-ray Machines

Recognising that early X-ray machines, e.g. 'Coolidge tubes' (10-150 kV) [1, 12, 13], were limited due to their inability to handle deep seated tumours, early research was focused on developing high voltage X-ray apparatus [51, 52]. One of the first serious advances to take place was the introduction of the so called 'X-ray cannons' (200-300 kV) in the 1920s; such devices allowing sufficient penetration to deal with deep seated tumours. However, it was not until the development of megavoltage X-ray apparatus that radiotherapy became a successful technique for the treatment of cancer. The first megavoltage X-ray machines appeared in the late 1930s, and a small number of radiotherapy centres were equipped with installations operating in the 300 kV-1 MV range [2, 12, 13]. Such devices were huge, in particular the X-ray tube at St. Bartholomew's Hospital, London, which remained in operation from 1944 to 1960, was 30 feet long and weighed some 10 tons [51, 52]. The size and price of these machines was such that only a few selected hospitals were able to be equipped.

It was the introduction of telecobalt megavoltage γ-rays, Cobalt 60 (Co60) (≈ 4 MV) [2], that revolutionised radiotherapy from the 1950s up to the early 1980s. Indeed Co60 units were very simple to use and extremely robust, as apart from routine maintenance, the only intervention required was to change the radioactive Co60 source every five years [2]. The development of linear accelerators (or linacs), 3 - 50 MV [25, 26], with the increased penetration offered, and the rapid developments in computer technology prompted the replacement of the Co60s by linacs in many centres throughout the 1980s. In addition linacs may also be used in electron mode (power expressed in MeV as opposed to MV for photon mode). Note that the electron mode is used for treating superficial lesions, whereas the photon mode is used for the treatment of deep seated tumours. An operational linac which is in use at Walsgrave Hospital, Coventry, is shown in Fig. 1.2.

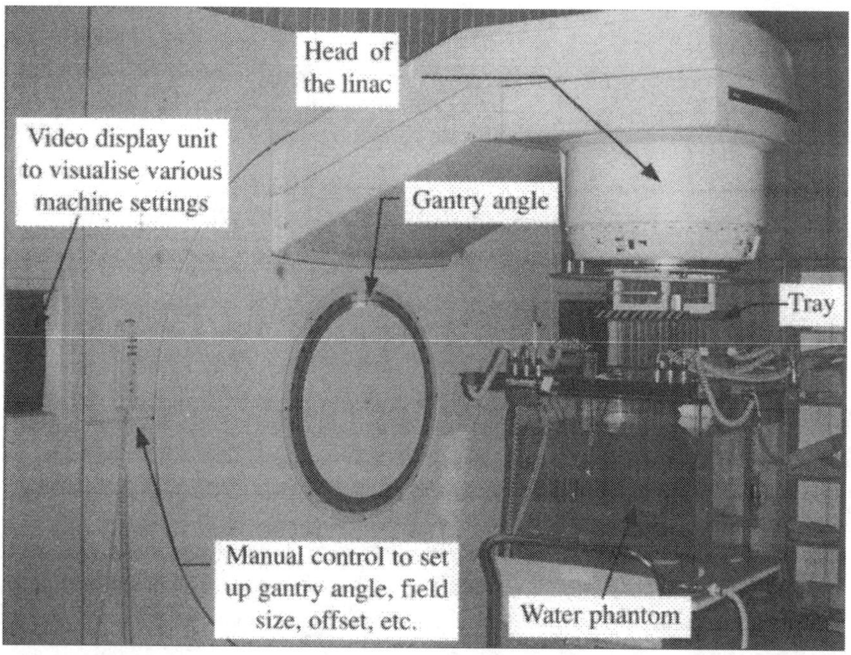

Fig. 1.2 Illustrating a 25 MV linac set up to perform measurements in a water phantom, courtesy of Walsgrave Hospital, NHS Trust, Coventry, UK

The X-ray beams delivered by linacs have several potential advantages and exhibit several interesting characteristics such as:

- higher energy beams which are less attenuated by human body structures than weaker beams
- much narrowed penumbras (see Chap. 2), which reduces the spread of the dose at the edge of the beam compared to the X-rays delivered by the famous 'X-ray cannon' [2, 12, 13], although the penumbra does begin to increase for beam energies greater than 10 MV due to secondary electrons
- maximum dose which, as opposed to early X-ray therapy apparatus, does not occur at the skin level but at a few centimetres below, thus producing the so called skin sparing effect [1, 2, 53] (see Chap. 2 and 3)

an increased distance between the X-ray apparatus and the patient, which allows more flexible and convenient direction of the beam, thus making possible the irradiation of a body from almost any angle. This is sometimes compromised by the use of additional devices fixed on the head of the linac.

Latest developments include the use of protons or heavy ions [3, 54, 55, 56] in order to improve the irradiation of deep tumours whilst sparing the dose to normal tissues. This is possible due to the different way in which these particles deposit their energy as dose compared with photons (X-rays).

Technological developments combined with advances in the field of computing, imaging and mechanics are providing clinicians and physicists with the tools necessary to produce high quality treatment. As such, the optimisation of radiotherapy treatment plans has become an important integral feature within the treatment of cancer. The next section reviews the various components involved in present day radiotherapy treatment planning procedures.

1.3 Radiotherapy Treatment Planning Procedures

As mentioned above, the use of external X-ray photon beams to eradicate malignant cells also affects healthy normal tissues and organs [2, 3, 4, 53]. As a consequence, radiotherapy is used when no other technique is practical or when cancerous cells show an increased radiation sensitivity compared to healthy tissues. The aim is, therefore, to deliver a suitably high radiation dose to the diseased tissues without exceeding radiation tolerances to the surrounding tissues; thus avoiding risk of complication [3, 4], whilst ensuring the total eradication of the disease.

1.3.1 Conventional Radiotherapy Procedures

Recommended radiotherapy procedures are issued by the International Commission on Radiological Units and Measurements (ICRU) to ensure that procedures are achieved repeatedly and qualitatively [24]. It involves determining the location, the extent, the stage and the shape of the tumour. According to this clinical information, the clinician may decide to use external beam therapy with a treatment prescription being issued. In some cases, additional data may be required from computed tomography (CT) or magnetic resonance imaging (MRI) scans for this planning stage of the treatment.

Making use of such information, regions of interest (ROIs), which influence the planning process, are delineated to describe the patient contours and the position and shapes of the organs. Such image segmentation is currently performed manually on a few selected CT slices. However, in order to make IMRT a clinical reality it is necessary to delineate the ROI on all CT slices. The latter prompts the need for automatic or semi automatic image segmentation, see [57] for example, where novel image segmentation techniques are used to segment whole CT sets automatically. A three-dimensional (3-D) reconstruction algorithm may then be used to visualise the ROIs.

According to the geometry of the ROIs and the clinical specifications, a provisional beam arrangement is selected by the treatment planner and the predicted dose distribution calculated. By manipulation of the beams, dose distribution predictions are compared in order to select an optimal treatment plan. This phase may be partially automated by making use of an algorithm, which calculates automatically the dose distribution resulting from a particular beam setting and varies one or two beam parameters, to find an acceptable distribution in the target. However, in most cases the treatment planner or the physicist is required to provide and compare alternative solutions. Therefore, an acceptable solution, that may not be the optimal solution, is determined in a semi empirical manner based on experience and good practice involving several trials of various alternative solutions [2, 3]. Note that in order to reduce the time required to evaluate each candidate treatment plan, a simplified beam model may be used by the treatment planning system for this initial stage of the planning process. Once an optimal plan which is clinically acceptable has been selected, an accurate calculation is computed with a full beam model for clinical approval [3, 24]. Each treatment plan proposed by the treatment planner and the physicist is verified by the clinician. The treatment is delivered with the radiation therapy machine set in accordance with the plan specified.

In order to determine the outcome of the treatment it is necessary to adopt a procedure of 'patient follow up' and subsequent analyses of the results. Note that this latter stage may take up to several years, as a relapse may occur several years after the initial treatment. Usually five years survival is considered as a cure [2, 3, 4, 24].

In this work attention is focused on the planning stage that is referred to as radiotherapy treatment planning (RTP).

1.3.2 Radiotherapy Treatment Planning

In order to be able to deliver high quality treatment via external beam radiation, a substantial effort is required by the treatment planners, medical physicists and clinicians planning and simulating the treatment options. Treatment planning can be defined as the process of entering the patients' details such as geometrical information concerning the shapes of the ROIs together with the diseased region from anatomical information provided by various imaging facilities such as CT or MRI scans [2, 57, 58]. It also involves the determination of beam arrangements (location, shape, compensation) that results in the generation of a clinically acceptable treatment plan.

To ensure the reproducibility and the accuracy of the treatment plans quantitative and qualitative procedures are developed. Automating part of the optimisation process such that it is operator independent is one such procedure. This includes the development of RTP quantitative assessment methods, which are not solely based on the visual inspection of isodose plots resulting from the optimisation, but on dose area histograms identifying the dose intensity received by different regions (see Chap. 4, 5 and 6) .

1.3.3 Automated Treatment Planning: Review of the Developments

From the late 1950s to the mid 1980s RTP was a two-dimensional (2-D) operation for both dose calculation and display [3, 4]. The dose calculation algorithms were based on tissue-air-ratio and scatter-air-ratio, making use of 2-D look-up up tables of measured dose and empirically derived functions to fit the measured dose [59]. These models are for particular beam apertures under ideal conditions. For some special cases such as, for example, compensators inserted on a tray fixed to the treatment machine head (see Fig. 1.3), special measurements are required as the models did not provide reliable predictions.

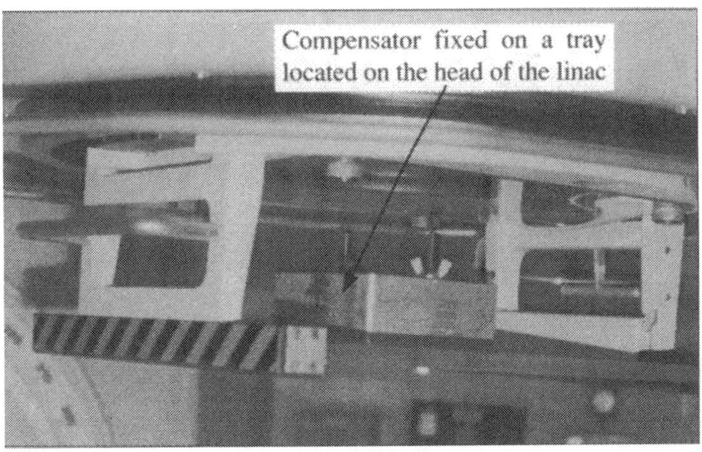

Fig. 1.3 Compensator used for research purposes at Walsgrave Hospital, NHS Trust, Coventry, UK (courtesy of Walsgrave Hospital, NHS Trust, Coventry, UK)

Dose distributions are traditionally represented with 2-D isodose curves. Conventionally 2-D RTP is carried out on what is referred to as the 'mid-field slice'. This is actually a plane through the patient in the middle of treatment volume and in which all beams lie. With this approach, only limited beam arrangements can be planned for, using coplanar beams with the possible addition of beam modifiers such as wedges or lead blocks. With this arrangement, the treatment planner is required to determine an acceptable plan by making use of a forward planning strategy, which is basically an experienced trial and error procedure based on good practice. Although tumours are likely to have irregular shapes, it is common practice to 'box in' treatment areas using cubic or rectangular parallelepiped or cylindrical volumes [2, 4, 24].

Today the use of CT and the development of visualisation software has enabled modern RTP systems to display the ROIs and to visualise the path of the beam in 3-D [35, 56, 60]. Furthermore 3-D dose calculation algorithms enable the treatment planner to assess more accurately a wider variety of field shapes and intensity modulated X-ray beams [3, 4, 56]. The increase and widespread availability of computer power has led to the use of sophisticated optimisation techniques to determine the optimum beam configuration for the goals set by the clinicians [3, 4, 35, 60, 61]. Whereas a conventional manual 2-D RTP system relies mainly on visual inspection to assess a treatment plan, modern automated RTP systems are not only used for dose display purposes, but also to produce optimised plans that fulfil the clinicians' prescriptions. They are also able to display predicted performances in terms of dose area (2-D) or dose volume (3-D) histograms [3, 24, 62, 63].

1.3.4 Beam Compensation Techniques

Radiotherapy requires the production of a uniform dose over the planning target area (PTA). In order to do so, devices to modify the beam intensities have been developed. Beam intensity modulation is considered to be an important contribution towards improving the physical selectivity of the treatments delivered by external beams. Similar to traditional wedge compensating methods, in-field intensity modulation can be produced by static techniques, such as patient specific transmission blocks and compensating filters [38, 39, 40, 41, 42, 43], or dynamic techniques such as dynamic collimation apparatus [44, 45, 46, 47, 48, 49, 50]. This section briefly reviews some of the techniques that are currently in use and some of which are currently under development.

Static Beam Compensation Techniques. Traditional radiotherapy makes use of fixed wedge shaped beam compensation devices, also named wedge compensators, see Fig. 1.4. These compensators can be inserted directly in the head of the treatment machine or positioned on a tray in the beam path. Wedges are differentiated according to their 'wedge angle'. The British Standard Institution (BSI) [64] defines the wedge angles as the slope of the isodose contour at standard measurement depth (i.e. 10 cm depth) [24, 64], see Fig. 1.5. The wedge angles most commonly used are 15°, 30°, 45° and 60° [4]. Such devices are discussed in more detail in Chap. 6.

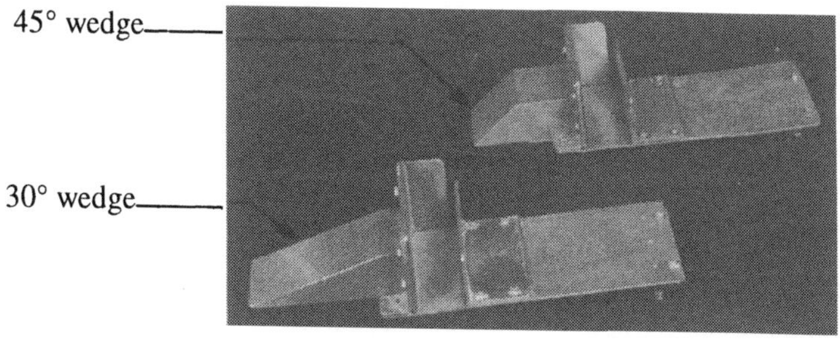

Fig. 1.4 30° and 45° wedges that can be inserted into the head of the linear accelerator to modulate the beam intensity across the field into a wedge shape (courtesy of Walsgrave Hospital, NHS Trust, Coventry, UK)

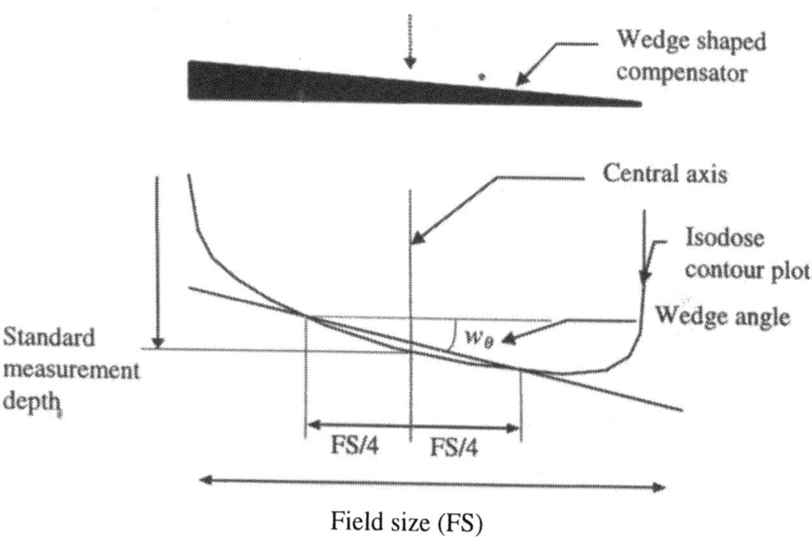

Fig. 1.5 Illustrating the concept of wedge angle

Compensators, made from radiation attenuating material, inserted in the beam path or positioned against the patient skin were first used to compensate for patient contours. These compensators were usually made of low density materials such as wax and referred to as 'missing tissue compensators' [3, 38, 40, 42, 65]. Transmission blocks have also been used to correct for inhomogeneities [2, 39, 40, 66] and high density material compensating filters have been used to modulate the beam intensity [39, 40, 41, 42]. In this work, high density low melting point alloys are used to allow the design of relatively thin compensators whilst being able to deliver highly modulated beams. These patient specific compensators operate on the same principle as wedges. Therefore they are robust, reliable, easy to use and reproducible. They can be placed at a distance from the patients' surface, so the skin sparing effect is retained. In addition, it is possible to design such compensators using sophisticated optimisation algorithms such that they provide a means of producing conformal treatment, thus improving the physical selectivity of the overall plan. Indeed, it is against this background that the work presented in this monograph is based.

Dynamic Beam Compensation Techniques. Dynamic beam compensation techniques, such as dynamic wedges and the high resolution multi-leaf collimators (MLCs), move mechanical parts (leaves) automatically during the treatment. These devices were developed in the late 1970s and early 1980s. However, it is only since the beginning of the 1990s, with the improvement of computer controlled machines and the use of modern control techniques, that their potential to routinely modify the beam fluence (or in-field beam intensity) has been realised [3, 67, 68, 69, 70].

For the dynamic wedge, one field diaphragm moves across the field during irradiation and in this way a wedge field profile is produced. With the MLC, the multiple lead or tungsten leaves are moved under computer control during the course of the treatment, either continuously or discontinuously where, for each leaf incremental position setting, only an incremental portion of the total dose is delivered [3, 4, 48]. However, although MLCs have been shown to be able to deliver intensity modulated beams [49, 50], they are nowadays mainly used as flexible secondary collimation systems; with each of the leaves being positioned at the beginning of the treatment to conform to the beam's eye view, or shape of the target [2, 3, 4, 31, 32, 33], see Fig. 1.6.

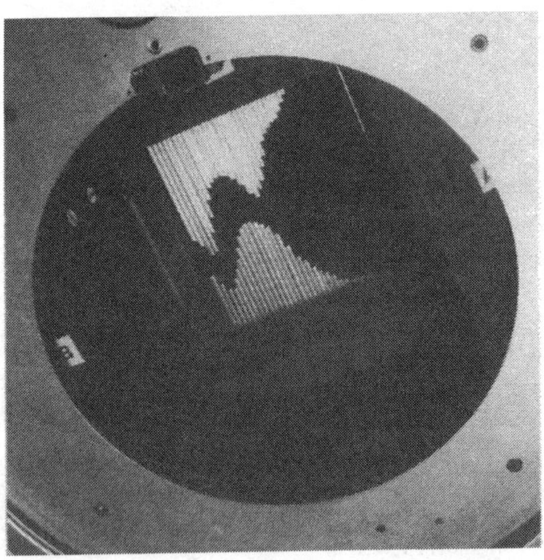

Fig. 1.6 Example of MLC, seen from the patient view point, used to shape a field according to the beam's eye view of the diseased region (courtesy of Elekta)

MLCs have been shown to be an efficient substitute to beam shaping and blocking [32] which has been performed since the 1960s with specially shaped lead blocks inserted into the beam path to reshape the target from the beam's eye view [4]; thus avoiding the irradiation of critical structures, such as the eyes.

The ability of such collimation machines to produce automatically a wide range of beam shapes and beam modulations are considered to be more flexible than static techniques that require the manufacture of patient specific blocks or compensators [3, 4]. In addition they have the potential to be automatically updated to account for the change in patient position and condition. Therefore dynamic techniques are potentially more flexible and faster than static techniques. Their main drawback is the amount of computer power and the complexity of the software required to deliver dynamic treatment safely. Also, in comparison to static techniques, MLCs are more complex to set up and rely heavily on the reliability and correct functioning of mechanical devices and computer software to drive the leaves. A problem inherent to MLC design using 'tongue-and-groove' or 'stepped edge' to reduce leakage between adjacent leaves, is the underdosage of as much as 10% - 15% of thin regions along the boundaries of the leaves [71]. In [71] it is shown that the 'tongue-and-groove' effect could be minimised by synchronising pairs of leaves so that they complete irradiation simultaneously. The latter, however, may add further constraints on the beam profiles which can be delivered. To overcome the above problems and to exploit the advantages offered by both static and dynamic methods, a number of centres make use of MLCs to automatically provide field shaping, i.e. spatial modulation, combined with compensators to provide a simple and robust beam modulation device [2, 3].

Alternative Compensation Techniques. Other non uniform beam delivery systems are also under development. One particular method makes use of the concept of tomotherapy [72, 73, 74]. It aims to include both treatment delivery and treatment assessment apparatus in the same machine; thus making on line monitoring of treatment delivery a clinical reality. The beam delivery part of the machine is inspired from an electro-mechanical device previously developed, known as MIMiC® [75, 76, 77], see Fig. 1.7. The beam exiting the MIMiC® is divided into two thin slices of 1 cm, and each slice is subdivided into 20 smaller beams. The treatment is delivered slice by slice, with the MIMiC® system rotating around the patient to treat two slices at a time. Each leaf can move quickly during the treatment, thus producing intensity modulated beams. However, for successful results, this technique requires an almost perfect immobilisation technique and minimal movement of internal body structures. This may explain why it has so far only been used favourably, when compared to stereotactic radiosurgery, with the head of the patient being screwed onto a stereotactic frame to ensure a quasi perfect immobilisation [78].

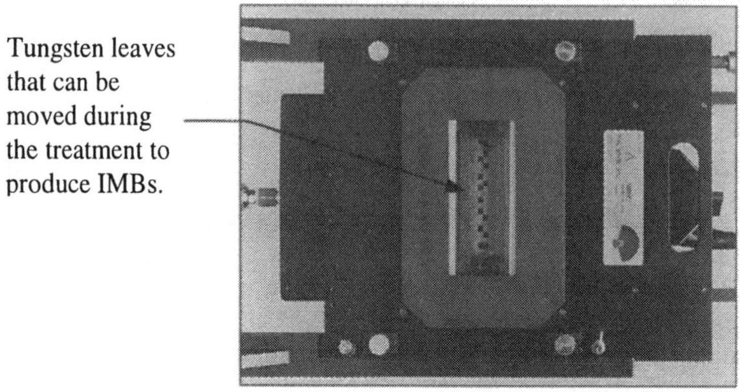

Fig. 1.7 MIMiC® as seen from the patient (courtesy of NOMOS Corporation)

Treatment Delivery Techniques. There are two different categories of treatment delivery:

- Radiation can be delivered continuously by a method known as rotation therapy, where the linac is rotated around the patient during the treatment [3]. Note that this technique was the first dynamic therapy developed [60].
- The linac is moved to a number of set positions around the patient which have been predetermined in the planning process. At each position an intensity modulated beam is delivered [3].

The first technique utilises the benefits of rotation therapy in that the relative dose received by the target is much higher than the dose received by the other tissues. The disadvantage of this method is that most of the healthy tissue receives a dose of radiation. The second technique is simpler, with multiple static beams. It can spare particular regions and takes less time to deliver. In this work the second technique is considered as only an approach involving multiple static beams can lend itself for use with compensators.

1.4 Background to the Optimisation of Radiotherapy Treatment Plans

The particular aspects of RTP dealt with in this monograph are the optimisation of:

- coplanar beam orientation
- wedge angles and beam weights

– intensity modulated beams.

The first two problems can be considered as combinatorial optimisation problems [4, 10], whereas the last problem has been referred to as an 'inverse problem' [3, 4, 5].

1.4.1 Traditional Approach to Manual Optimisation

The optimisation process followed by physicists can be described as a forward knowledge based iterative process [3, 4]. In order to determine the best plan, the treatment planner will typically investigate several different beam configurations. These methods are well known and a skilled treatment planner, making use of well known standard plans, can arrive to a solution relatively quickly. Nevertheless, due to the limited number of trials together with the reliance on well known beam configurations, the resulting plan, although clinically acceptable may neither be optimal nor repeatable.

The use of modern beam shaping techniques such as universal wedges, dynamic wedges or in-field intensity modulation devices involve a much larger number of variables. This makes it more difficult for an optimal solution to be achieved manually. This multiplication of interactive variables influencing the outcome of a treatment has prompted the need for computer assisted decision making to help clinicians select the best clinically acceptable solutions. The latter has prompted the need to translate clinical factors into mathematical expressions that reflect the patients needs [3, 4, 79].

1.4.2 Consideration of Region of Interest

In order to optimise radiotherapy treatment plans, it is necessary to identify all the ROIs (see Fig. 1.8). In terms of cancer treatment, the most important structure is the diseased region. In order to be able to compare treatment in different centres, guidelines have been issued by the ICRU Report 50 [24] on standard procedures to define the region to be treated. This region is referred to as the planning target volume (in 3-D RTP), denoted PTV, or the planning target area (in 2-D RTP), denoted PTA. The PTV is a geometrical description defined to select appropriate beam sizes and beam arrangements, taking into consideration the effect of all possible geometrical variations and inaccuracies in order to ensure that the prescribed dose is actually absorbed by the clinical target volume denoted CTV. This means that the PTV should account for the movement of organs during the course of the treatment, which may take many weeks, together with the variations that may occur in the patient positioning. Therefore the PTV depends on the treatment technique, the anatomical site of the disease, and the type of immobilisation or positioning procedure adopted. The CTV is the tissue volume that contains a gross tumour volume, denoted GTV, and/or sub-clinical microscopic malignant diseases, which have to be eliminated to ensure total eradication of the disease. The GTV is the palpable, visible or demonstrable extent and location of the malignant growth which is the region where most of the diseased cells are located. In this work, one slice at a time is considered, therefore the regions to be treated are referred to as areas instead of volumes (see Fig. 1.8). For example the PTV becomes the PTA. For a concave PTA it is necessary to determine a point that is within the PTA and for which the dose is required to be ideal. Guidelines given in ICRU Report 50 [24] propose that a point of reference should be located at the isocentre of the GTA (see Fig. 1.8). For convex PTA the isocentre usually corresponds to the centre of gravity of the GTA.

The other regions that are required to be outlined are the organs at risk (OARs), i.e. the spinal cord and the rectum for pelvic region. The main bone structures are also required to be taken into account for changes in radiation attenuation. Other healthy tissues (OHT), which are also taken into account are all the tissues not considered as belonging to the PTA or the OARs. For example in Fig. 1.8, the OHT includes the muscles, fat and bones in the pelvic region.

Note that all CT slices are conventionally viewed from a patient's toe (i.e. along the toe to head axis). Consequently the patients' right is on the left of the Figure.

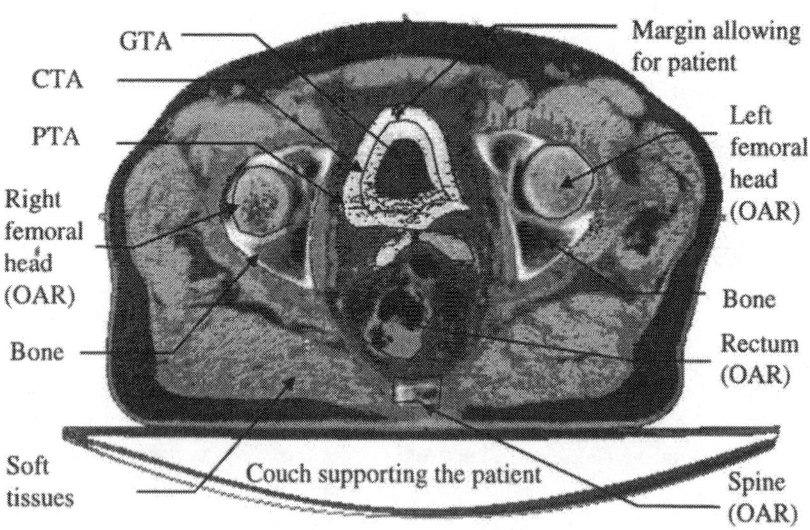

Fig. 1.8 CT slice of a pelvic region with manual delineation of the bones, the organs at risk, the target (allowing for marginal spread and patient movement)

1.4.3 Notion of Objective Function

In order to be able to produce a solution, it is necessary to describe the treatment process in mathematical terms. In particular, in order to quantify and compare the relative benefits of a given treatment plan over another, it is necessary to assess the efficacy of each plan by making use of an objective function. An objective function describes in mathematical terms the aims of an optimisation process. In radiotherapy, the ultimate aim is to cure the patients or at least provide the patients with some form of relief and improved quality of life. Due to the progressive effect of radiation, effects of treatment are required to be assessed over a period of many years; recalling that a five year survival is taken as a cure.

The concept of quality of life is becoming more and more important in assessing the outcome of a treatment for a terminal or incapacitating disease [35, 79], although it is not at all easy to define or quantify the meaning of quality of life. In order to determine the 'best' treatment for a particular patient several variables are required to be taken into account. Some of the most important considerations are, the stage of the disease and the age and the fitness of the patient. These considerations should be included in the prescription stage. By making use of such information an adequate prescription can then be determined and subsequently planned.

Biological models have been developed to model the 'real' objective of radiotherapy, which is to deliver a suitable dose to the cancerous cells whilst minimising the risks of complication due to an overdosing of healthy tissues, in particular organs at risks [2, 3]. This involves the biological modelling of cell response to irradiation [80, 81, 82]. Biological models are given in terms of tumour control probability (TCP) and normal tissue control probability (NTCP). TCP gives a measure of the likelihood of controlling the disease and, therefore, achieving an eradication of all the cancerous cells. NTCP provides an indication of the risk of complication due to the dose received by some specific structures for which the NTCP are calculated. Biological modelling is currently favoured in the United States, but due to the difficulty in assessing such models, more traditional assessment methods, based on dose requirements, remains the accepted standard in Europe [3]. A recognised advantage of biological models is their ability to take into account dose-volume relationships. Recent research carried out in parallel with the work presented in this monograph, see Bortfeld *et al* [83], has shown that it is possible to implement clinically relevant objectives using physical criteria, with the dose volume requirements implemented as constraints. In the work presented in this monograph it is assumed that an appropriate prescription may be defined in terms of a dose specification only. The need to achieve a particular dose is then expressed via individual objective weightings as opposed to constraints, see Chap. 4. Although this demonstrates the use of the objective function concept; the guidelines given by the ICRU Report 50 [24] for biologically based models could also be used for comparison.

1.4.4 Objective Based Dose Criteria

Treatment is presented in terms of the amount of dose radiation necessary to irradiate a particular cancerous region. Depending on the nature of the disease and the overall condition of the patient, different dose levels are specified to the isocentre of the GTV. This maximum dose level is normalised to 100% and used as a reference for the treatment plan. The objectives for the PTA, OAR, OHT are now given.

Planning Target Area. The latest guidelines of the ICRU for improved standardisation of prescriptions require the dose in the PTA to be high and uniform. The dose should be normalised at the centre of the PTA to 100% with the dose elsewhere within the PTA being in the range $100 \pm 5\%$. Achieving this first objective should ensure that the disease is cured. Nevertheless as highlighted by Moore in [35] 'cure at any cost' is no longer an acceptable approach to treatment. Quality of life after treatment is important.

Organs at Risk. In order to improve the quality of life by reducing the side effects of the treatment, OARs have to be spared as much as possible. The sparing of an OAR at all cost requires the beams to be positioned such that they do not overlap over a particular organ. In practice the clinicians may wish to preserve the spine in the treatment of neck cancer, or one of the lungs when the other lung is being irradiated to treat a diseased lung. However, in cases where a small irradiation is unavoidable, this amount needs to be minimised.

Other Healthy Tissues. The dose delivered to the other healthy tissues (OHT) must also be minimal. High dose regions in the OHT receiving more than the dose prescribed to the isocentre of the PTA are referred to as hot spots (HS) [24]. In this work, the definition of HS is extended to include that which is considered as a high dose region, although the dose may not be as high as the dose received by the PTA. HS usually occur within the beam paths, in low depth regions, close to the skin. They arise due to the nature of the radiation attenuation in human tissues, where the dose initially escalates before decreasing exponentially with depth. The usual method of reducing HS is to increase the number of beams involved in a plan, thus decreasing the maximum dose delivered by any one beam. In this way the treatment planner attempts to produce plans with HS covering similar volumes and at similar dose levels.

Definition of Objective. In order to express mathematically the objective, the CT slice is superimposed onto a matrix grid which makes use of Cartesian co-ordinates. As such, each element of the grid is denoted d_{ij} so that the section is represented by an n by m matrix grid. Subscript notation is used to distinguish between elements that lie in the PTA, OAR and OHT regions such that $d_{PTA_{ij}}$, $d_{OAR_{ij}}$ and $d_{OHT_{ij}}$ denote the desired dose corresponding to the elements at the ith row and j^{th} column of the PTA, OAR and OHT respectively.
Making use of the above notation, the desired dose in the PTA is defined as:

$$95\% \le d_{PTA_{ij}} \le 105\% \tag{1.1}$$

where a dose of 100% represents the normalised desired dose in the isocentre of the GTA. The desired dose in the OAR is defined as:

$$0\% \le d_{OAR_{ij}} \le x_1\% \tag{1.2}$$

where $x_1\%$ is the maximum dose allowed (should the dosage be unavoidable) and depends on the OAR considered. In the work considered here it may be as low as 20%. In the case of OHT, the desired maximum dose may be expressed as:

$$0\% \le d_{OHT_{ij}} \le x_2\% \tag{1.3}$$

where $x_2\%$ is normally chosen such that $x_2\% \ge x_1\%$. Note that all percentages are in terms of the desired dose at the isocentre (or centre) of the GTA.

Having established the desired dose for the three ROIs, all the procedures (with the exception of beam orientation) for optimising the RTP in this monograph are based upon minimising some cost function which involves the difference between the desired dose and that predicted using a given beam configuration. Defining the predicted dose as $\tilde{d}_{PTA_{ij}}$, $\tilde{d}_{OAR_{ij}}$ and $\tilde{d}_{OHT_{ij}}$ the objective is to seek a solution to a minimisation problem of the general form:

$$J_{(\mathbf{d}-\tilde{\mathbf{d}})} = \alpha\left[\mathbf{d}_{PTA} - \tilde{\mathbf{d}}_{PTA}\right]^{\mathrm{T}}\left[\mathbf{d}_{PTA} - \tilde{\mathbf{d}}_{PTA}\right] + \beta\left[\mathbf{d}_{OAR} - \tilde{\mathbf{d}}_{OAR}\right]^{\mathrm{T}}\left[\mathbf{d}_{OAR} - \tilde{\mathbf{d}}_{OAR}\right] + \gamma\left[\mathbf{d}_{OHT} - \tilde{\mathbf{d}}_{OHT}\right]^{\mathrm{T}}\left[\mathbf{d}_{OHT} - \tilde{\mathbf{d}}_{OHT}\right] \tag{1.4}$$

where the quantities $\mathbf{d}$ and $\tilde{\mathbf{d}}$ with the appropriate subscripts are vectors corresponding to the d_{ij} and $\tilde{d}_{ij}$ elements in the PTA, OAR and OHT, respectively, and α, β and γ are scalar weighting factors for each of the ROI.

Whatever optimisation technique is used, the final implemented solution will necessarily attempt to simultaneously satisfy an objective of the form (1.4).

The RTP optimisation problem is clearly a multi-objective optimisation problem with expression (1.4) being a weighted sum of the objectives involved in RTP based on dose criteria. Ideally the solution of this problem would require each of these objectives to be solved simultaneously. However, in most cases it is not possible to do so and a trade-off between the objectives has to be determined. Such a trade-off is in general chosen empirically prior to the optimisation but the disadvantage of this approach is that it may produce an optimal solution which is not clinically acceptable. In order to overcome this problem a novel use of the concept of Pareto optimality in the context of RTP is investigated (see Chap. 5 and 6).

1.5 Optimisation in Radiotherapy: A Brief Review

Optimisation of radiotherapy treatment aims to provide the treatment planner with a tool to semi-automate RTP procedures and generate candidate treatment plans. It is not aimed to replace the clinician, who is ultimately responsible, but should provide tools to facilitate the assessment of the proposed treatment plans in a more efficient way. In this monograph three optimisation problems in the context of RTP are investigated. These are: determining the optimum number and orientation of the beams; determining the optimum combination of beam intensity (or weight) and wedge angle; and determining the optimum set of intensity modulated beams to produce conformal therapy.

1.5.1 Optimisation of Coplanar Beam Orientation

The first step in any planning procedure is for the treatment planner/clinician to select the number and orientation of the beams. Then, during planning, the beam gantry angles, i.e. the angle made by the line passing through the beam CAX and the vertical axis, may be slightly modified to improve the overall dose distributions. By making use of good practice and empirical knowledge the clinicians are able to find appropriate beam settings relatively quickly. In addition, it has been shown that the influence of an optimum beam orientation on the dose distribution in the target is relatively small compared to other factors such as the beam shape [3, 4, 84] and the in-field intensity modulation. This perhaps explains why the beam orientation problem has received only a limited attention in the literature [3, 27, 29, 30]. In traditional radiotherapy the limited number of beams involved in a plan enables the clinician to determine manually, based on experience, the best beam orientation more efficiently than computerised methods. But with the increased complexity of treatment plans, especially in conformation therapy, and the accompanying increased number of beams involved in a plan, the task of determining the 'best', in some sense, beam orientation may become difficult and/or tedious. The problem is illustrated in Fig. 1.9, which shows a schematic representation of the path of two beams in relation to the gantry angle of the treatment machine.

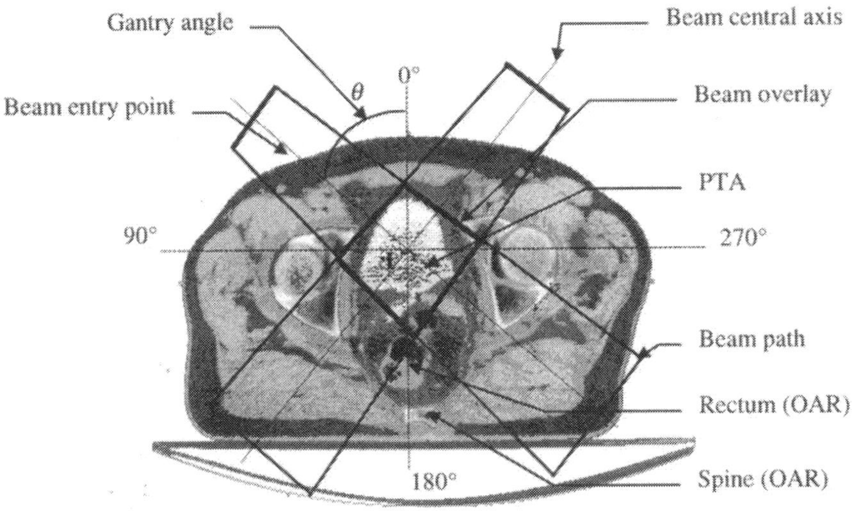

Fig. 1.9 Optimising the beam orientation

A number of researchers have attempted to solve the beam orientation problem, but due to computational problems and the fact that improvements obtained were marginal compared to manual optimisation techniques, such solutions have been slow to emerge into the clinical environment, see for example [27, 29, 30]. In Chap. 6 the beam orientation problem is revisited and a novel approach is proposed which makes use of hybridised genetic algorithms.

The approach adopted in this work is similar to that of Bortfled [27] in that a stochastic or random search based method, namely a genetic algorithm (GA), is used within an iterative process to determine the optimum beam orientation. The main disadvantage of search techniques that are based on a random process, such as GAs or simulated annealing (SA) is that they require a large number of function evaluations. In order to reduce the time required to evaluate a particular set of beam orientations a novel geometrical formulation of the coplanar beam orientation problem, that does not require the pre-calculation of the so-called dose calculation matrix for each new beam angle, is proposed. The proposed approach, which is inspired from the process followed by treatment planners to determine acceptable beam orientations, is detailed in Chap. 6.

One of the main aspects of novelty in this work builds on an approach to multi-objective optimisation in RTP, where all the objectives are considered simultaneously by obtaining a set of non dominated solutions; also referred to as the Pareto optimal set [1, 11, 85], see Chap. 6. Alternative acceptable solutions can then be selected from the set of candidate solutions with a decision maker (DM) that can adapt its preference to that of a particular clinician.

1.5.2 Optimisation of Beam Weight and Wedge Angle

Classical radiotherapy makes use of wedges and simple conformal radiotherapy, which shape the beams to the beam's eye view of the PTA, and may also utilise wedge shaped compensator devices. The optimisation techniques are required to find the 'best' combination of beam intensity, or beam weight, and wedge angle, where both beam weight and wedge angle can be restricted to standard known incremental values. Beam weights are usually given in terms of percentage depth dose, where a weight of 100% produces a beam for which maximal dose is 100%.

Essentially the problem may be viewed as shown in Fig. 1.10, where the beam weight is represented by the thickness or height of the compensator on the central axis; in this case three beams are considered.

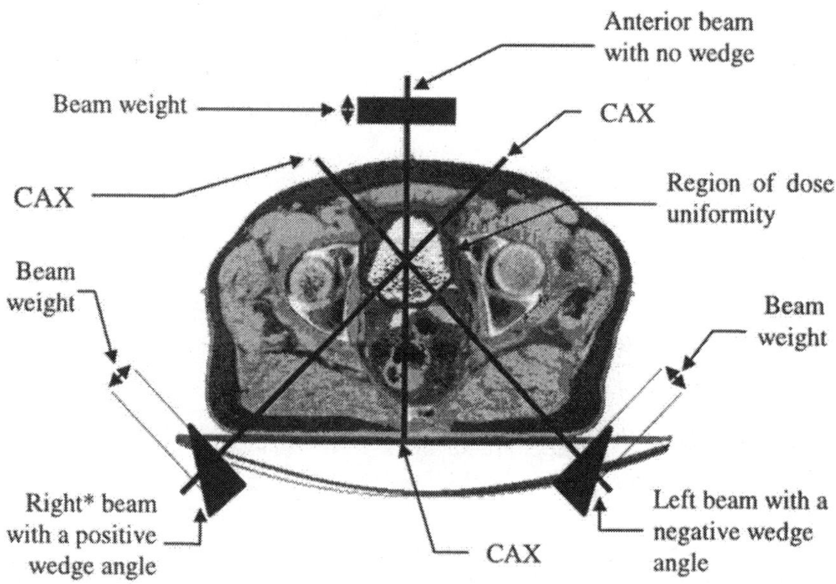

Fig. 1.10 Optimising wedge angles and beam intensity or weighting (traditional beam arrangement for a three field plan)

*Note that with reference to Fig. 1.8, the beam shown on the left of Fig. 1.10 is known as the right beam, i.e. right of the patient.

There are a number of techniques available to produce wedge shaped fields. The simplest technique involves the use of wedge shaped compensators with a particular wedge angle, i.e. having a 30, 45 or 60 degree wedge angle. Alternatively use can be made of the so called universal wedge [86] (see Chap. 6) which can produce any wedge angle by combining an open field with a fixed wedge field. The problem is then to determine the beam weights for both the open and the wedged fields. In this monograph, in order to develop a procedure that does not depend on the technique used to produce a wedged field, beam weight and wedge angles are considered as two independent variables.

The optimisation of beam weight/wedge angle can be viewed as a combinatorial problem, where the aim is to find the optimal combination of beam weight and wedge angle. Several heuristic search techniques have previously been used to solve this problem [86, 87, 88, 89, 90, 91]. The method of SA has been used successfully in [36, 37, 88] to determine the optimal beam weight combination. However, the high computational effort required by traditional SA made it a slow process, which makes it unrealistic for use in RTP systems. In order to overcome this problem, fast simulated annealing (FSA) has been applied to the beam weight optimisation problem [37, 38, 87], and it has been shown to converge up to ten times faster than SA. Constrained simulated annealing has also been used to find a feasible solution for a set of constrained beam weights [87]. The constraints can be modified so that if early convergence occurs, the set of constraints is relaxed, i.e. the minimum beam weights are reduced so that new possible solutions can be attained. An approach which assumes a homogeneous media has been proposed [90] which enables wedge angles and wedge orientation to be selected. The approach provides a conceptual basis to solve the problem using geometry but may be limited especially when dealing with inhomogeneous media. GAs have been used for beam weight optimisation and compare favourably to SA [91]. In this work a multi-objective GA, similar to the one used in [30, 92] has been hybridised to exploit problem specific features of the RTP problem.

1.5.3 Optimisation Methods for in Field Intensity Modulation

In the absence of beam intensity modulation it is possible to produce plans that conform to convex tumour geometrical shapes, usually achieved by making use of a large number of beams. However, it has been shown [3, 4, 5, 7, 8] that in order to produce a plan which is fully conformal with a concave PTA, intensity modulated beams (IMBs) are required. The optimisation of IMBs is considered to be a more complex problem than the optimisation problems previously described. The main difference is that the clinicians' prescriptions for conformation therapy are much more demanding than they are for traditional radiotherapy, where only a limited number of beam modifiers are available. In conformation therapy, the clinician is able to prescribe much more complex treatment plans by making use of information provided by modern imaging techniques together with other clinical information. For example in treatment of prostate cancer, the PTV usually covers all the prostate volume, which may be concave with the rectum, which is an organ at risk, in its near proximity. Making use of traditional beam compensation techniques it is not possible to produce a treatment plan that conforms to such a concave PTV, whereas with field intensity modulation uniform irradiation is possible [3, 4, 49, 50, 67, 68, 69, 70]. The concept of IMB is illustrated in the schematic diagram of Fig. 1.11 in which the standard wedge shaped compensators of Fig. 1.10 are replaced by more complex shaped profiles.

The problem of determining an optimal set of intensity modulated beams (IMBs) from clinicians' prescriptions is referred as the inverse problem [1, 2, 3, 36, 68, 69, 74, 93, 94, 95, 96, 97] and this is a central feature of the work reported in this monograph, see Chap. 4. Essentially, the inverse problem in RTP is that of working back from a dose prescription to obtain the optimal set of intensity modulated beams. Some of the techniques that have been proposed by other workers in the field are briefly reviewed here.

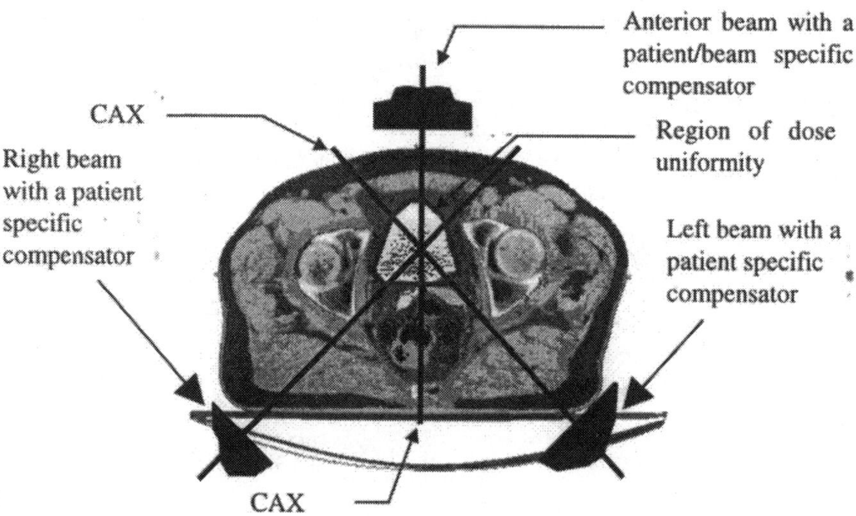

1

Several techniques have been used to solve the inverse problem in radiotherapy. Most of these techniques require the dosage delivered at specific dose calculation grid points to be represented as a set of linear functions of the IMBs. For convenience, in previous work, the problem has been formulated such that the number of IMBs equals the number of dose calculation grid points [3, 5, 7, 68, 98, 99, 100]. A dose calculation matrix which describes the interactions of the radiation with the body structure is pre-calculated such that the dose is given by the product of this dose calculation matrix with the vector describing the IMBs. In order to solve for the IMBs it is only necessary to determine the inverse of the dose calculation matrix and to multiply this by the dose prescription arranged into a vector form. In practice it has been found that due to sparsity, i.e. a large number of null valued elements in the matrix, it is not practical to invert such a dose calculation matrix and an approximation of the inverse of the dose calculation matrix is required to be formulated [3, 5, 8, 101]. Several of these approximations have been reviewed in [71]. Use of such approximations leads to a mismatch between the real effect of the dose irradiation and that modelled in the optimisation process. Consequently most of the previous methods verify the dose distribution obtained from the optimisation procedure with a more accurate model for the purpose of display, and hence final verification. A brief summary of the previous proposals to solve the inverse problem are as follows:

Brahme [5] in 1988 proposed the steepest descent algorithm together with multiple pencil beams, with a dose calculation matrix and a Hessian matrix being approximated by the product of an identity matrix with a scalar. (The approach was demonstrated in the 2-D case.)

Lind [101] in 1990 proposed a 'modified gradient algorithm' with the Hessian matrix approximated by an identity matrix. The use of spatially invariant electron beams does not allow any account for inhomogeneities. (The approach is applicable to 3-D but has only been demonstrated in 2-D.)

Bortfled [7] in 1990, made use of 'filtered projection' to give a good initial starting point for the 'scaled gradient projection' algorithm which is then used to refine the solution given in terms of individual pencil beams. In this approach, inhomogeneities were not taken into account and the scattering effects were 'approximately' calculated using an equivalent field method. Note that the optimisation algorithm used to refine the solution approximated the Hessian matrix by a diagonal matrix [2, 6, 70]. (Although it is possible to make use this method in 3-D, results were presented for the 2-D case only.)

Holmes [8, 72, 75, 99, 102] in 1993 used an iterative filtered backprojection technique with individual pencil beams where the Hessian matrix was approximated by the identity matrix and the inverse of the dose calculation matrix is simplified so that only the primary contribution is considered. Similar to the previous approach, inhomogeneities and beam divergence are not taken into account. Furthermore, 3-D optimisation is achieved by optimising sequentially 2-D slices [102].

Yuan [100, 103] in 1994, has used Bayesian and maximum entropy optimisation with individual pencil beams accounting only for the beam primary contribution in homogeneous medium. (The approach is used only for 2-D.)

The approach followed in this work differs from that of previous researchers in that the solution is formulated as a hybrid approach involving iterative least squares and genetic algorithms, see Chap. 6. Essentially the first phase of the optimisation makes use of iterative least squares to solve the inverse problem assuming parallel beams. This makes use of a new beam model which takes into account both primary and scatter radiation, and allows for inhomogeneities to be taken into account in the primary (see Chap. 2 and 3). The second phase makes use of a divergent beam model (again involving primary and scatter and the ability to handle inhomogeneities) in which the solution is adapted to the new beam model and refined by forward solving techniques using GAs. In this way the problem of mismatch between the optimal dose and that achieved in reality is reduced. The approach is briefly outlined in Sect. 1.5.5.

Remarks: The approach developed in this work can be demonstrated for both homogeneous and inhomogeneous media and the scatter is also taken into account in the determination of the inverse problem. This alone should ensure that a better theoretical solution can be obtained from the RTP simulation software developed.

The practical aspects of the implementation of the 'theoretical' solutions are dealt with in Chap. 6.

Initially the divergent beam model was not considered suitable to be used in the solution of the inverse problem by iterative least squares (ILS); but used in conjunction with GAs in a forward solving optimisation procedure. As the work progressed, the need for a hybrid approach became apparent and a method which made use of both parallel beam and divergent beam models with ILS and GAs was developed (see Chap. 4 and 5). This forms the basis of the experimental work reported in Chap. 6. The aim of the hybrid approach was to demonstrate that a solution obtained with a particular beam model could be adapted to another more realistic beam model with a GA. However, after completing the experiments, it became apparent that the divergent beam could also be adapted for use with ILS.

1.5.4 Need for a Matrix Based Beam Model

In this section consideration is given to the basis and principle of the beam model developed in Chap. 2 and 3, for solving the inverse problem. It is useful at this stage to consider a CT slice normal to the patient head to toe axis as shown in Fig. 1.12.

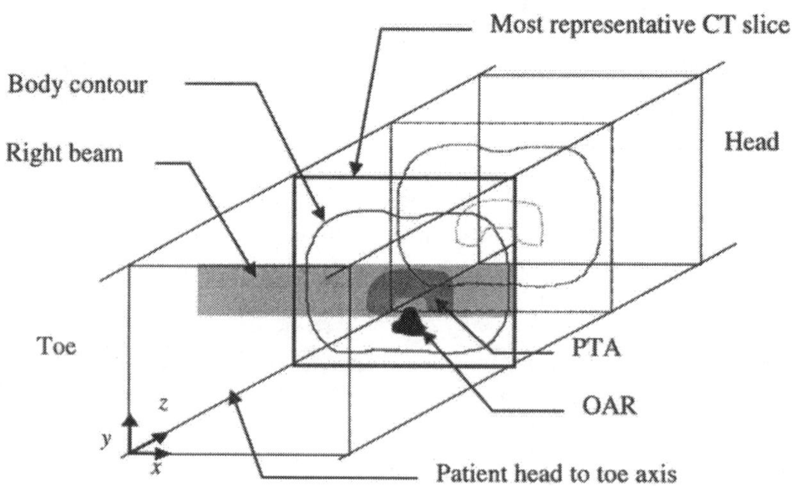

Fig. 1.12 Illustrating the orientation of the CT slice within the patient

Making use of a grid structure an elemental representation of a beam dose matrix may be shown as in Fig. 1.13.

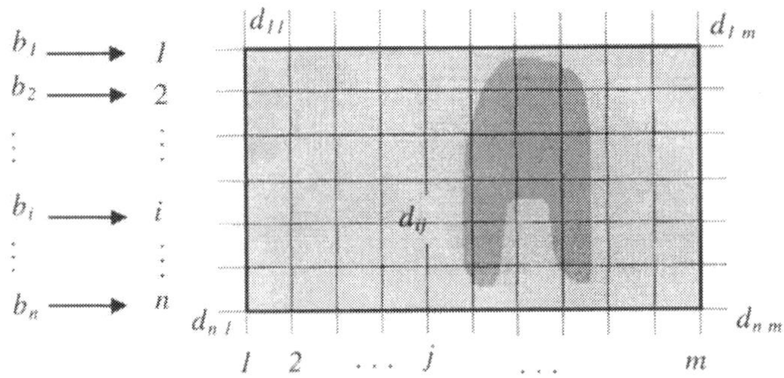

Fig. 1.13 Illustrating a beam dose matrix

The effect of multiple beams is shown in Fig. 1.13, which illustrates two beams at right angles from which the total dose matrix, denoted **D**, is obtained by summing the two (in this case) individual beam dose matrices onto the reference grid.

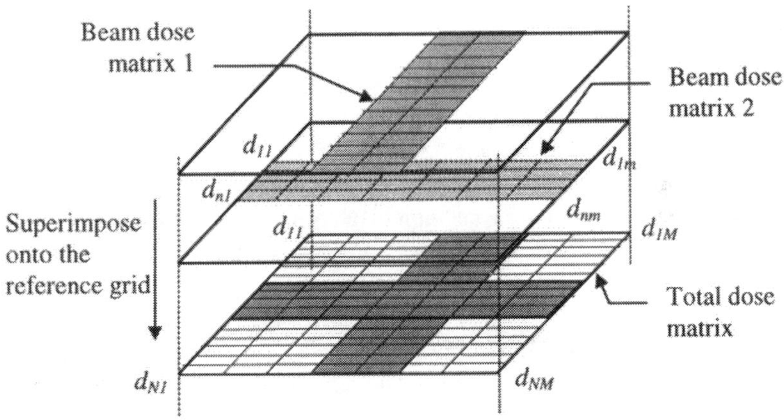

Fig. 1.14 Illustrating the superposition involved in the summation of two beams in the case where grid elements of the beam dose matrices correspond to those of the reference grid

The effect of the two beams is obtained as the summation of the two beam dose matrices within the reference grid. Note that whilst the total dose matrix necessarily involves elements that are outside the body structure (see Chap. 2 and 3), these elements are not taken into account in the optimisation procedure. Note that for the reasons of ease of manipulation in the calculation, the beams are assumed to enter at the left side, with the reference grid (representing the patient) being rotated to allow for the correct beam entry. (In reality the beams rotate and the patient is immobilised.) Note that the elements of the total dose matrix $\mathbf{D} = \{d_{ij}\} \in \Re^{N \times M}$ represent the individual dosages to the elemental cells. To illustrate the basic concept, consider a single beam entering from the left $\mathbf{b} = [b_1 \ldots b_n]^T$, $\mathbf{b} \in \Re^n$ which relates to the dose delivered in each cell $\{d_{ij}\}$. Defining the grid area as a partitioned vector $\mathbf{d} = [d_{11} \ldots d_{n1} \; ; \; d_{12} \ldots d_{n2} \; ; \; \ldots \; ; \; d_{1m} \ldots d_{nm}]^T$, i.e. $\mathbf{d} \in \Re^{n.m}$ where each partition corresponds to a column in the beam dose matrix; it is possible to formulate the problem such that

$$\mathbf{d} = \mathbf{\Phi}\,\mathbf{b} \tag{1.5}$$

where $\mathbf{\Phi} \in \Re^{(n \times m) \times n}$ is known as the beam dose calculation matrix. Equations of the form (1.5) can be constructed for each beam i=1...k in the plan, see Chap. 3.

1.5.5 Proposed Hybrid Approach

The approach to optimisation of RTP in this work consists of a two stage optimisation process. The first stage involves the use of a novel parallel beam model (introduced in Chap. 2 and 3) together with a scheme of iterative least squares (ILS) to solve for the inverse problem. Having obtained a solution(s) using this approach, the second phase of the optimisation procedure makes use of a more realistic divergent (or fan) beam model to adapt the theoretical solution found by ILS to the practical case using GAs. The advantage of ILS is that it can reach an acceptable solution in a very small number of iterations. The disadvantage is that such an algorithm requires the objectives to be expressed in terms of a quadratic objective function. Such a formulation may not be optimal to describe the clinical requirements. In addition it requires a particular formulation of the beam model, that is a simplified representation of the actual beam delivery system. GAs, on the other hand are much slower that ILS, typically requiring at least ten to a hundred times more iterations [104]. However, they have the advantage of being flexible in the sense that they can accommodate any objective function and are not constrained to quadratic objective functions only. Moreover, such an approach does not impose any particular requirement on the beam model, only that a model is able to calculate a dose distribution from a set of candidate intensity modulated beams. In this work the advantages of the two algorithms are combined in that the speed of ILS enables an acceptable dose distribution to be determined which forms an initial set of solutions for the GA to perform a local search to improve the solutions obtained with the simplified beam model. GAs offer a problem independent solving framework [1, 10, 30], that can be exploited to advantage by making use of a more realistic beam model. Such a model could include the beam divergence as well as taking into account the limitations of the physical beam modulation systems, to adapt the theoretical solution found by ILS to the real world. The provision of an initial starting point for the GAs reduces the number of iterations required to fine tune the solution with a physically more realistic beam model. The overall operation of the approach is illustrated diagrammatically in the flow diagram of Fig. 1.15.

Note that in this monograph the principle of this approach is investigated with a 2-D based beam model. However by considering multiple slices the approach could be used to achieve a solution for a 3-D dose calculation problem.

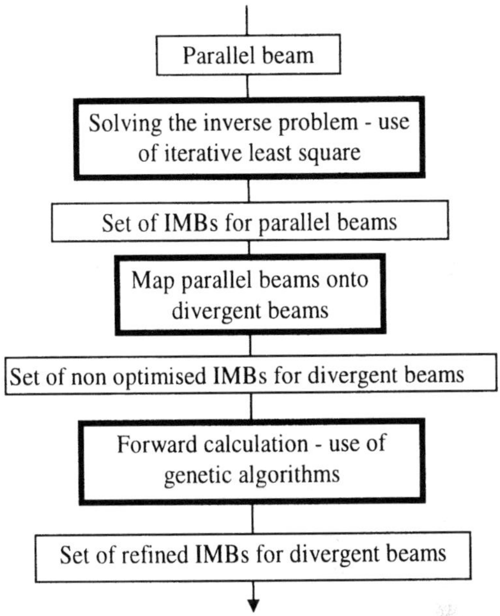

Fig. 1.15 Schematic representation of the hybrid approach involving ILS and GA techniques

1.6 Concluding Remarks

This Chapter has given a brief overview of the developments that have taken place in the field of radiotherapy treatment. By considering initially a historical review of some of the early pioneering research, the Chapter has followed the steps leading to the present day state of the art technology. The advances that have been witnessed in the area of X-ray apparatus and radiotherapy treatment machines have taken place in parallel with rapid developments in microcomputer hardware and software technology. Such advances are evident in medical image processing, thus allowing for a better definition, realisation and verification of radiotherapy treatment.

Various methods for achieving conformal therapy have been briefly introduced and justifications for making use of patient specific compensators have been presented. The principle of the approach, which is currently the subject of research and development between Coventry University and Walsgrave Hospital NHS Trust, Coventry, has been discussed.

The aims of radiotherapy treatment have not changed and are firmly focused towards the total eradication of cancerous tissues, whilst at the same time sparing healthy tissues. Technological advances today facilitate the use of more sophisticated equipment and correspondingly more complex treatment plans. Whereas traditional radiotherapy could be administered using manual methods of optimisation, the demands arising from the use of more complex treatment plans has prompted the need for automatic (or semi automatic) approaches to solve the overall optimisation problem. In the latter respect, an overview of some of the developments in optimisation of the so called inverse problem have been reviewed and the principle of an alternative hybrid approach reported in this monograph has been outlined.

CHAPTER 2
BEAM CHARACTERISTICS AND PRELIMINARY MODELLING CONSIDERATIONS

2.1 Introduction

The aim of a radiotherapy treatment planning (RTP) system is to determine clinically acceptable dose distributions prior to the physical delivery of the treatment. It has been seen in Chap. 2 that present day RTP systems offer the possibility to make use of three dimensional (3-D) information to determine clinically acceptable plans. However there is not yet a RTP system that offers optimisation algorithms to determine automatically optimal 3-D treatment plans. One of the main reasons is that the algorithms developed to date are still too slow to operate in the demanding clinical environment in a cost effective manner. This is due to the fact that in general the algorithms are required to perform many hundreds if not thousands of iterations which are highly computer intensive due to the complexity of evaluating a 3-D dose distribution with a full 3-D beam model. As a consequence most of the optimisation algorithms developed have used simplified beam models to perform most of the optimisation. Such optimisation is carried out prior to the implementation of an optimised solution into a system with a full 3-D beam model. This principle has been adopted within the Peacock RTP software of NOMOS Corporation, in which use is made of the filtered back-projection algorithm developed by Holmes *et. al.* [8, 71, 74, 76, 99]. Essentially, a starting point to the optimisation in [99] is initially determined, with subsequent refinements being obtained through the use of simulated annealing (SA) together with a more sophisticated beam model.

2.2 Need for an Appropriate Model Structure

When attempting to obtain a useful model of any process it is necessary to have a clear understanding of how the model is to be used; since such information will undoubtedly influence the choice of the model. The RTP system model, introduced here and developed in Chap. 3, is aimed at demonstrating novel optimisation procedures that can, at a later stage, be implemented within an existing RTP system in a clinical environment. As such, the beam model, which is a central feature of the RTP simulation software, emulates the features of the two dimensional (2-D) RTP system [105] used for clinical routine treatment at Walsgrave Hospital when the work was carried out. This model provides a platform that can be used to demonstrate novel optimisation schemes on classical RTP problems such as the optimisation of the combination of wedge angles and beam weights. Nowadays, however, the most demanding optimisation problem is that of working back from a prescribed dose distribution to the optimum set of intensity modulated beams (IMBs) to solve the inverse optimisation problem (see Chap. 4). Recognition of the nature of the problem prompts the need for a matrix based beam model [106] (see Chap. 3), which lends itself ideally to optimisation and control of the IMBs [106, 107, 108]. In the model that is developed, each beam is divided into elemental pencil beams, each of which represents an element of the beam that can be modified by an elemental compensator. In this way, the compensators, which are inserted into the beam path as shown in Fig. 2.1, produce intensity modulated irregularly shaped beams to conform to the treatment specified by a clinician.

Traditional models that have been developed to achieve conventional treatment in RTP systems have only needed to express a forward relationship between standard beam input, such as wedge shaped beam profiles, and the beam dose distribution. Most of these models make use of look-up tables where measured dose values are stored for a particular beam configuration. Based on the look-up table results, intermediate values may be obtained by interpolation. Such models make use of the so called tissue-air-ratio (TAR) and scatter-air-ratio (SAR) [59] or differential-scatter-air-ratio (DSAR) [109, 110, 111].

The beam models that are used to solve the inverse problem are required to account for irregular beam profiles and, as a consequence, the traditional look-up table model approach cannot be used. The most popular approaches make use of pencil beam models. Some beam models previously developed to solve the inverse problem construct a dose calculation matrix that gives the total dose distribution from a given set of intensity modulated beams. This leads to sparse dose calculation matrices that have to be inverted making use of iterative process and approximations [3, 5, 8, 72].

In the approach proposed in this monograph, the model developed includes scatter and correction for inhomogeneities; with the resulting model being used in the optimisation process, see Chap. 4, 5 and 6. The beam model which is introduced here and developed in Chap. 3 considers each beam independently, thus a dose calculation matrix is constructed for each beam involved in the treatment plan. The resulting individual beam dose matrices, are n by m rectangular matrices with $n < m$. These matrices are used to solved for the individual beam weights (or intensities) by making use of the pseudo inverse [9]. The overall problem may be considered to have been divided into N_{Beam} smaller problems, where N_{Beam} is the number of beams. Note that the solution of the overall problem involves an iterative procedure to reduce the error via repeated calculation of the pseudo inverse, with the successive individual solutions being superimposed in order to obtain an iterated overall solution.

As well as solving the IMB problem, the developed model can also be used to optimise traditional RTP plans involving the determination of the optimal combination of wedge angles and beam weights.

As opposed to simplified beam models, previously used for optimisation purposes [5, 36, 37, 68, 97, 100], the pencil beam model developed here accounts for radiation scatter, inhomogeneities, penumbra, and patient contour correction. By including such physical characteristics into the model, which is used to solve the optimisation problem, the discrepancy between a full and fairly accurate beam model and a beam model developed for optimisation purposes only is significantly reduced. As a consequence, the solution should then be more readily realisable.

The beam model is aimed to replicate a system in which the input is a given set of IMBs and the output is a dose distribution. In this work the IMBs represent the beam profile at the point of equilibrium; that is the point at which the dose is maximum. This point is located between 1 cm and 4 cm (for photon beams) below the patient surface [25, 26]. The modelling of the compensator requires the observed beam profile at the point of equilibrium to be linked to compensator geometry (i.e. in terms of thickness) that would produce such an IMB. This procedure is illustrated in Fig. 2.1.

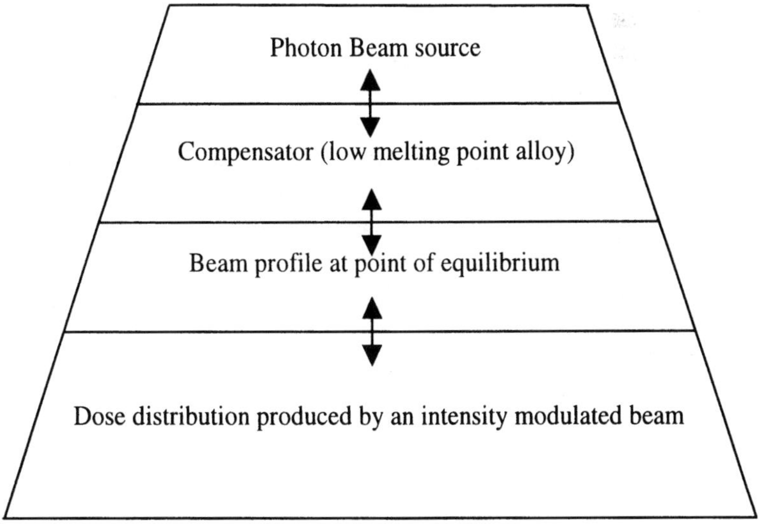

Fig. 2.1 Diagrammatic illustration of the approach used to calculate the beam dose distribution from an original compensator profile and vice versa

2.3 Preliminary Physical Considerations

This section introduces several terms and concepts that are required in order to follow the semi-empirical mechanisms that have been used to formulate the beam model in Chap. 3. First a brief overview of the most relevant characteristics of the behaviour of a photon beam produced by a linear accelerator is given.

Linacs produce high power X-ray photon beams by generating pulses of electrons through an electron gun. The generation of electrons is synchronised with the energising of the electron accelerating waveguide that is used to progressively accelerate the electrons from about 41% of the velocity of light to a velocity which is close to that of light. In the last part of the waveguide the energy is transformed as a gain in the mass of the electrons [53].

In order to prevent electrons from diverging use is made of coaxial coils. In addition two pairs of beam steering coils located at each end of the waveguide can be used to steer the overall electron beam through the system to ensure that it is correctly centred. Linacs, being able to rotate their head around the patient to deliver radiation, are required to make use of a beam bending chamber which is surrounded by a strong magnet to direct the electrons onto an X-ray target to produce photons. The photon beam generated passes through a primary collimator and a flattening filter (see Sect. 2.3.1) prior to being shaped according to specification by a secondary collimation device, and, where available, a multi-leaf collimator (MLC), see Fig. 2.2. The collimator enables the shaping of square or rectangular fields whilst the MLC can produce fields that conform to the 'beam's eye view' of the target. The beam's eye view is the shape of the ROIs as seen from the source.

The small source dimension (X-ray target), compared to the beam aperture, also referred to as a diaphragm, produces a divergent photon beam which passes into the patient (see Fig. 2.2).

A tray, which can be fixed to the head of the machine, is traditionally used to provide support for blocking materials inserted into the beam path to shield OARs, such as the eyes, from radiation. In this work it is used to position and fix compensators manufactured from a low melting point alloy. The tray is usually made of perspex and pierced with holes through which screws can be inserted in order to immobilise the compensators, thus enabling the linac head, and therefore the compensator, to rotate around the patient.

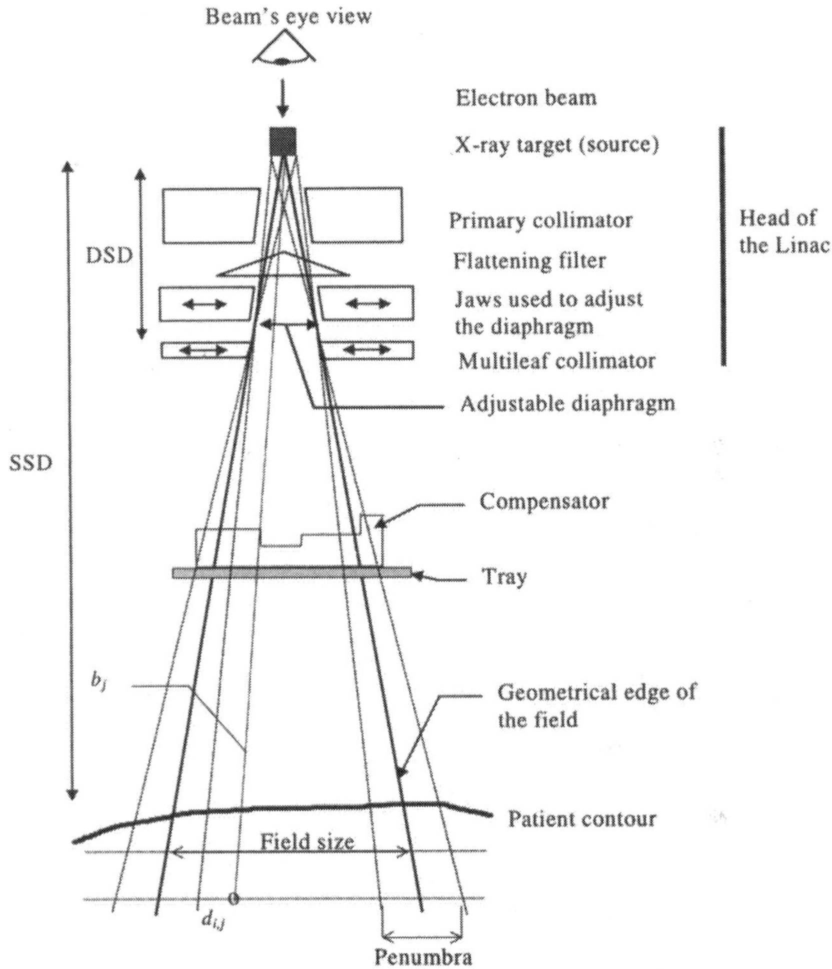

Fig. 2.2 Schematic diagram representing the main physical characteristics of a linear accelerator used to produce intensity modulated fields via patient specific compensators fixed on a tray

2.4 Typical Beam Characteristics

Prior to undertaking the modelling exercise in Chap. 3, it is worthwhile considering some of the salient features which characterise a photon beam.

2.4.1 Photon Beam Central Axis Characteristics

Photon beams are characterised primarily by their central axis percentage depth dose (CAX %DD), which describes the dose at any point along the central axis of the radiation field. The dose is normalised such that the maximum dose denoted d_{max}, which occurs at a depth denoted x_{max}, for a given beam, often referred to as the point of equilibrium, is 100%; i.e. CAX %DD at x_{max} is normalised to 100. The absorbed dose measured in a water phantom* is observed to rise with increasing depth near to the surface following beam entry up to the point of equilibrium, located at x_{max}, where x_{max} = 1.5 cm for the 6 MV beam and 3.5 cm for a 25 MV beam considered in this work. This is due to the population of charged particles flowing toward the point of maximum dose [53]; this region being known as the build-up region. This progressive build up of the dose as depth increases results in a reduction in the amount of radiation received by the skin, thus creating the so called skin sparing effect. Beyond the build up region (i.e. for depth greater than x_{max}) the CAX %DD curve is found to decay exponentially [26, 27, 53, 112]. (In practice, other factors such as the field size and the presence of blocking material in the beam path have an influence on the dose level on the central axis [112].) The main factor influencing the dose on the central axis, however, is the beam energy.

In this work the CAX %DD is modelled independently for the build up region and the exponential decay region thus ensuring that the skin sparing effect is taken into account in the calculations. The CAX %DD has been found experimentally to take the following form:

- Build up region: $x < x_{max}$,

$$\text{CAX \%DD}(x) = \beta_1 e^{\beta_2 x} + \beta_3 \ln(x+0.1) + \beta_4 \tag{2.1a}$$

- Exponential decay region: $x \geq x_{max}$

$$\text{CAX \%DD}(x) = \alpha_1 e^{-\alpha_2 (x - x_{max})} + \alpha_3 x + \alpha_4 x^2 + \alpha_5 x^3 \tag{2.1b}$$

where x_{max} is the depth at which equilibrium occurs. For both the 6 MV and the 25 MV photon beams used at Walsgrave Hospital, the coefficients α_i and β_i which have been obtained from measured data using the simplex algorithm [113], are given in Tables 2.1 and 2.2 respectively.

---

* The measurements were performed at Walsgrave Hospital, NHS Trust, Coventry, to obtain the value of the exposure with use being made of two ionisation chambers (one for reference in air and one in the water tank). The resulting %DD was given by normalising the data with respect to the highest dose retrospectively to give d_{max} = 100%.

Table 2.1 Coefficients obtained to model the CAX %DD for a 6 MV photon beam

α_1	α_2	α_3	α_4	α_5	β_1	β_2	β_3	β_4
$1.01e^2$	$5.60e^{-2}$	$-2.04e^{-1}$	$9.29e^{-2}$	$3.82e^{-2}$	$1.78e^2$	$3.09e^{-1}$	$5.48e^1$	$-7.73e^2$

Table 2.2 Coefficients obtained to model the CAX %DD for a 25 MV photon beam

α_1	α_2	α_3	α_4	α_5	β_1	β_2	β_3	β_4
$9.93e^1$	$2.04e^{-1}$	1.52	$-4.26e^{-2}$	$3.00e^{-4}$	$6.79e^2$	$2.03e^2$	$4.84e^1$	$6.35e^2$

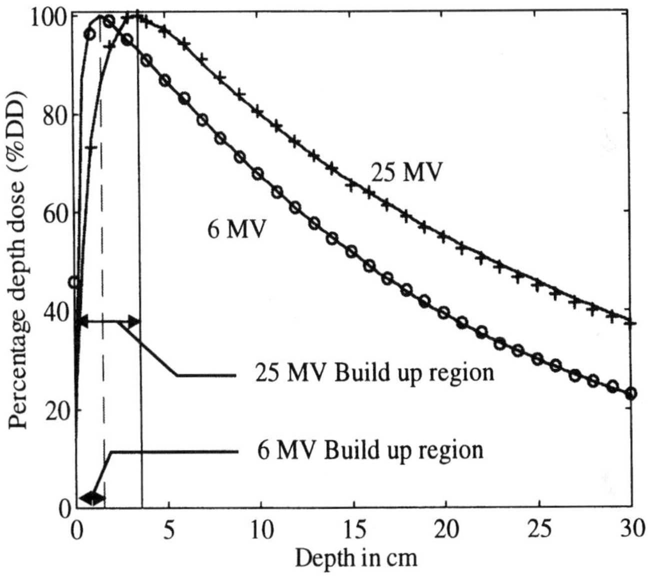

Fig. 2.3 Central axis percentage depth dose for 6 MV ('o' measured, '-' calculated) and 25 MV photon beams ('+' measured, '-' calculated)

In the development of the beam model it is important to ensure accuracy of the calculated dose at around a depth of $x = 10$ cm into the body since this is regarded by practising clinicians to be the depth at which particular attention must be focused. This depth is also referred to as the standard measurement depth [53]. The resulting model was found to satisfactorily match the measured data as shown in Fig. 2.3. It can also be observed in Fig. 2.3 that as the beam energy increases, x_{max} increases and the exponential decay reduces as a function of depth. The influence of beam energy in RTP is considered in more detail in Chap. 4 and 5.

2.4.2 In-Air-Profile

The dose across the beam is determined from the beam intensity measured in air. It is known as the in-air-profile (IAP). The IAP is a concave profile which results from the use of a flattening filter (see Fig. 2.2) in order to physically counteract the convex beam curvature which would otherwise occur. These flattening filters, which reduce the intensity of the beam in the centre of the field, usually overcompensate so that the beam entering the patient is characterised by slightly concave profiles at shallow depth, see Fig. 2.4, with increasingly convex profiles emerging due to scattered radiation as depth increases. In fact the flattening filter attempts to compensate both for the beam curvature resulting from the interaction of the electrons with the X-ray target and from the curvature of the beam arising from the Compton scattering effect [53, 114, 115], see Sect. 2.4.4; thus ensuring that the beam profile is reasonably flat at a depth of about 10 cm (depth at which the location of a tumour is likely in the pelvic region). Table 2.3 gives IAP data corresponding to a 25 MV beam used in the existing RTP system at Walsgrave Hospital. The IAP data were recorded at a distance of 100 cm from the beam source every 2 cm from the central axis up to a point situated at 16 cm on either side.

Table 2.3 Normalised IAP data for 25 MV photon beam used by the Bartec TPS V® RTP system at Walsgrave Hospital, NHS Trust, Coventry

Distance from the CAX (cm)	-16	-12	-8	-4	0	4	8	12	16
25 MV beam	1.025	1.030	1.020	1.010	1.000	1.010	1.020	1.030	1.025

Making use of data describing the IAP between 0-16 cm for the 25 MV photon beams, a polynomial approximation has been used to fit, in a least squares sense, a fourth order polynomial to the IAP data such that

$$\mathrm{IAP} = f_{iap}(y) = a_0 + a_1\,y + a_2\,y^2 + a_3\,y^3 + a_4\,y^4 \tag{2.2}$$

where y is the distance from the central axis and the coefficients of the polynomial approximating the IAP are given in Table 2.4

Table 2.4 Coefficients obtained to model the IAP for the 25 MV photon beam used by the Bartec TPS V® RTP system at Walsgrave Hospital, NHS Trust, Coventry

a_0	a_1	a_2	a_3	a_4
1.00	3.09e-3	-2.92e-4	-4.29e-5	-1.92e-6

Note that in order for equation (2.2) to be valid, the range of y is required to be bounded such that $|y| \leq 16$ cm. This permits a maximum field size of 32 cm by 32 cm which is considered to be sufficient for most cases.
The data from the Walsgrave RTP system and calculated IAP profiles for a 25 MV photon beam are given in Fig. 2.4.

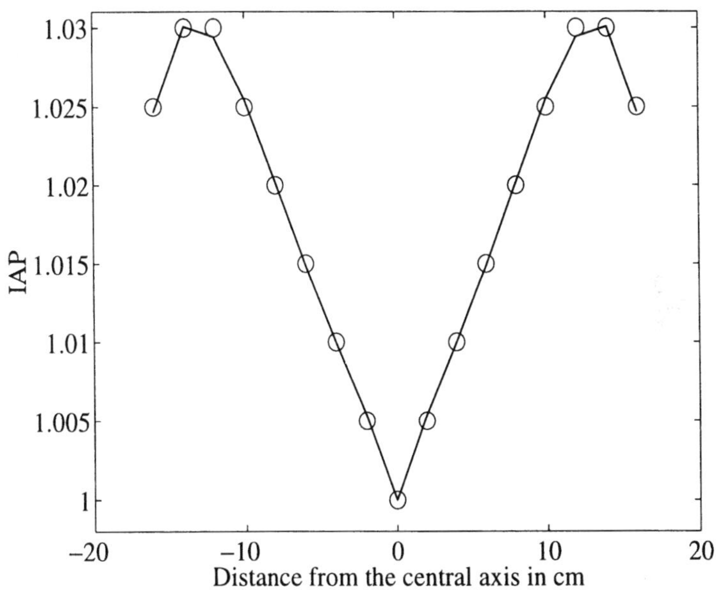

Fig. 2.4 Least squares fit of measured in-air-profile for a 25 MV photon beam (Measured data from by the Bartec TPS V® RTP system at Walsgrave Hospital, NHS Trust, Coventry are represented by 'o' and calculated by '-')

Note that the data stored in the RTP system used in Walsgrave Hospital NHS Trust are symmetrical although IAP may vary on a daily basis and may not therefore be exactly symmetrical. This asymmetry can be attributed to drift within the high voltage equipment used in the linear accelerators, e.g. electron gun and magnetron [53].

Applying the same technique to a 6 MV beam for data measured in the air, results in two fourth order polynomials P_l and P_2 (see equation 2.2). P_l, with coefficients a_{0l}, a_{1l}, a_{2l}, a_{3l} and a_{4l} given in Table 2.5, models the left side of the CAX. P_2, with coefficients a_{0r}, a_{1r}, a_{2r}, a_{3r} and a_{4r} given in Table 2.6, models the right side. Again y is bounded such that for P_l: $-16 \leq y < 0$ and for P_2: $0 \leq y \leq 16$ cm.

Table 2.5 Coefficients obtained to model the left hand side of the IAP for the 6 MV photon beam

a_{ol}	a_{1l}	a_{2l}	a_{3l}	a_{4l}
-1.07	3.31e-1	1.96e-1	-1.74e-2	3.37e-4

Table 2.6 Coefficients obtained to model the right hand side of the IAP for a 6 MV photon beam

a_{or}	a_{1r}	a_{2r}	a_{3r}	a_{4r}
-1.06	5.69e-1	6.33e-1	6.52e-2	1.82e-3

The measured and calculated IAP profile for a 6 MV photon beam are given in Fig. 2.5.

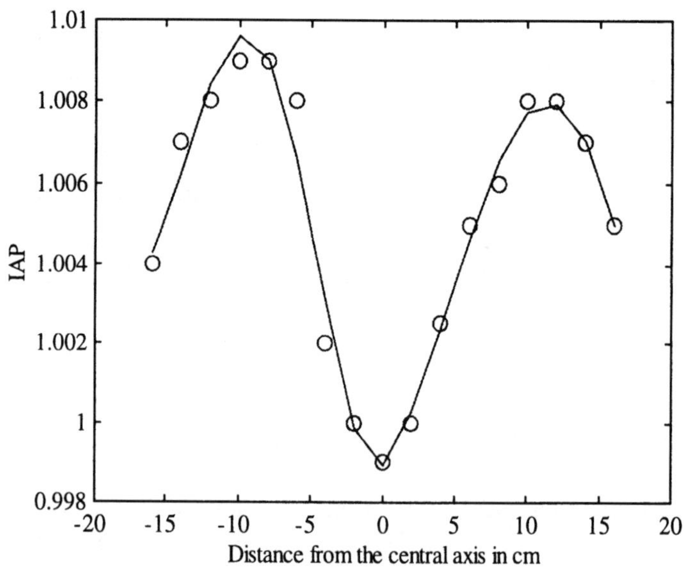

Fig. 2.5 Least square fit of measured in-air-profile for a 6 MV photon beam (Measured data from by the Bartec TPS V® RTP system at Walsgrave Hospital, NHS Trust, Coventry are represented by 'o' and calculated by '-')

2.4.3 The Penumbra

The penumbra is effectively the edge of the beam. In order to characterise the penumbra, its profile is modelled at a depth equal to x_{max}, i.e. corresponding to the point of equilibrium. The penumbra is dependent upon the distance of the diaphragm from the source (DSD), the source to skin distance (SSD) between the source and the patient surface, the beam energy and the depth of interest where the dose is specified. Typically, the dose in the penumbra region falls from 100% to a few % in 10 to 20 mm. The geometrical edge of the field defined by the solid fan lines (Fig. 2.2) passes through the centre of the penumbra region on each side of the beam as shown in Fig. 2.6. The 50% isodose line measured on a plane orthogonal to the central axis located at the depth x_{max} at which equilibrium occurs is used as a reference to determine the field size. The 50% percentage depth dose is marked by a dotted line in Fig. 2.6, which provides a visualisation of the width of the field at the point of equilibrium.

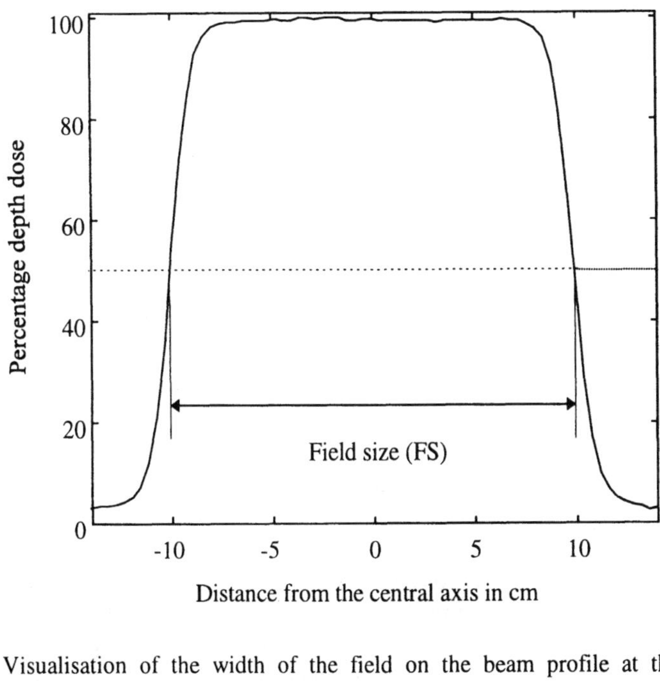

Fig. 2.6 Visualisation of the width of the field on the beam profile at the point of equilibrium (x_{max} = 1.5 cm for a 6 MV beam)

The intersection of the dotted line defining the 50 %DD with the beam profile at x_{max} on both sides of the CAX provides the width of the field or field size (FS). Traditionally, square or rectangular fields are used and field size is expressed in terms of length and width.

When use is made of MLCs or blocking materials, the shape of the beam is no longer a regular geometrical shape. In this case the field size is defined as the maximum length and width of the field. However, in order to determine the expected CAX %DD, equivalent square fields are required to be calculated.

Therefore, the dose delivered by the beam is usually given in terms of an equivalent square field [26, 27]. The reason for requiring an equivalent square field is that the CAX %DD, as well as the overall dose distribution, depends on the size of the field, i.e. the larger the field, the greater the beam intensity [107, 109, 110].

In this work penumbra characteristics for both the 6 MV and 25 MV beams have been modelled as fifth order polynomials which have been found to fit the measured data in a least squares sense, such that

$$Penumbra = f_p(y) = a_0 + a_1 y + a_2 y^2 + a_3 y^3 + a_4 y^4 + a_5 y^5 \tag{2.3}$$

where y is the distance measured from the geometrical edge of the field, i.e. a point located at a depth $x_{\max}$ where the dose is equal to 50% d_{max} is taken as the origin. The coefficients of the polynomials approximating the penumbra of the 6 MV and 25 MV beams for a 10 cm by 10 cm field are given in Tables 2.7 and 2.8 respectively.

Table 2.7 Coefficients obtained to model the penumbra for a 6 MV photon beam

a_0	a_1	a_2	a_3	a_4	a_5
$5.38e^{1}$	8.54	$-3.61e^{-2}$	$-5.20\ e^{-2}$	$1.27e^{-4}$	$1.32e^{-4}$

Table 2.8 Coefficients obtained to model the penumbra for a 25 MV photon beam

a_0	a_1	a_2	a_3	a_4	a_5
$5.20e^{1}$	9.18	$-2.08e^{-2}$	$-6.07e^{-2}$	$5.24e^{-5}$	$1.65e^{-4}$

Figures 2.7 and 2.8 show that a fifth order polynomial provides a sufficiently accurate fit to measured data for the penumbra regions corresponding to the 6 MV and 25 MV photon beams respectively.

Note that fifth order polynomials have been chosen in this work as they offer a good compromise between accuracy and over-parameterisation. To illustrate this, the sum of the squares of the error corresponding to the 3rd, 5th,7th and 9th order polynomials recorded for 15 data points considered using both the 6 MV and 25 MV beams are given in Table 2.9.

Table 2.9 Influence of the order of the polynomial on the accuracy of the model fit

Order of the polynomial	3	5	7	9
$\Sigma(\text{error})^2$ for a 6 MV beam	197.0	20.0	2.5	0.7
$\Sigma(\text{error})^2$ for a 25 MV beam	346.0	76.0	15.0	2.0

Note that the penumbra for a Co60 unit has previously been modelled with a seventh order polynomial [114].

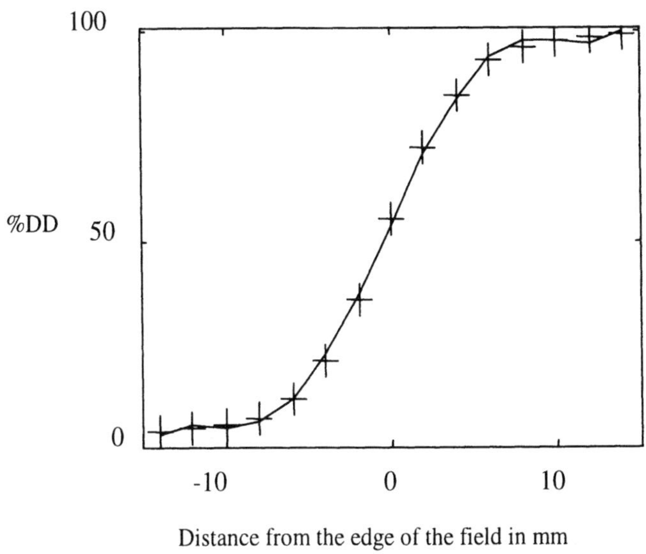

Fig. 2.7 Least square fit of the penumbra region for a 6 MV photon beam

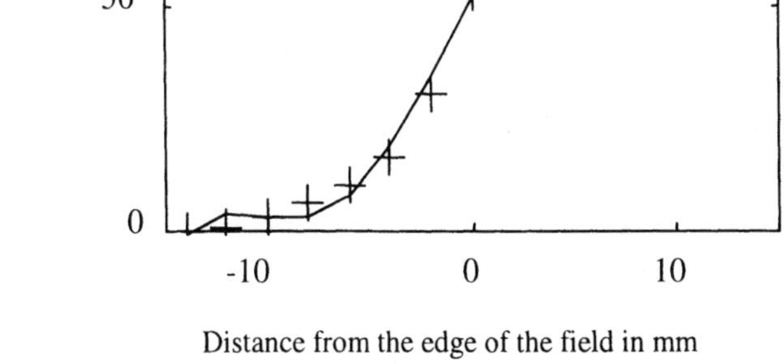

Fig. 2.8 Least square fit of the penumbra region for a 25 MV photon beam

2.4.4 Interaction of Photons with Matter

The interaction of electrons with the X-ray target produces more photons in the centre of the field than on the edges. This results in a beam that is convex after exiting the X-ray target. In order to compensate this effect, a flattening filter is used such that the beam entering the patient is usually flat or slightly concave. However, the interaction of photons with the body structures increases the beam curvature such that the beam profile convexity increases with depth. Photons interact with matter in a number of different ways which are fully detailed in [53]. The main types of interaction are the Compton effect, the photoelectric effect and the pair production [53]. The charged particles (i.e. electrons) produced from these interactions may then interact with matter to progressively transfer energy in the form of small Coulomb-force interactions [53].

External radiotherapy uses photon beams with a mean energy of several MV. For such levels of power, the dominant type of interaction between the photon beam and the human body structure is known as the Compton effect [53]. The Compton effect is characterised by the production of scattered photons and electrons by incident photons interacting with matter (see Fig. 2.9).

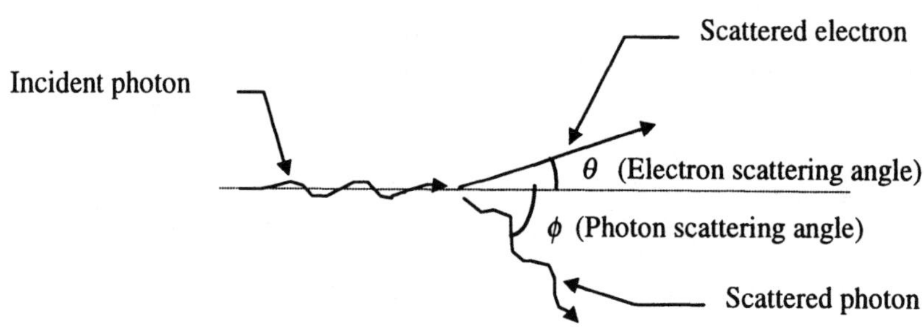

Fig. 2.9 Illustration of the Compton scattering caused by the collision of a photon with an electron, resulting in the production of a scattered photon and electron

The probability for scattered radiation to be produced in the forward direction is much higher than the probability of producing scattered radiation at any other angle [53]. This scattered radiation results in a beam curvature in the forward direction, increasing the percentage depth dose (%DD) at the centre of the field with respect to the dose on each side of the central axis (see Fig. 2.10). The beam curvature increases as the beam energy increases due to the increased number of photons produced in the forward direction.

As the radiation penetrates into the body structure it may be observed that the dose delivered in the region near to the central axis increases compared to the dose on the edge of the field creating increased beam convexity in the forward direction, see Fig. 2.10, which correspond to measured data for a 6 MV beam.

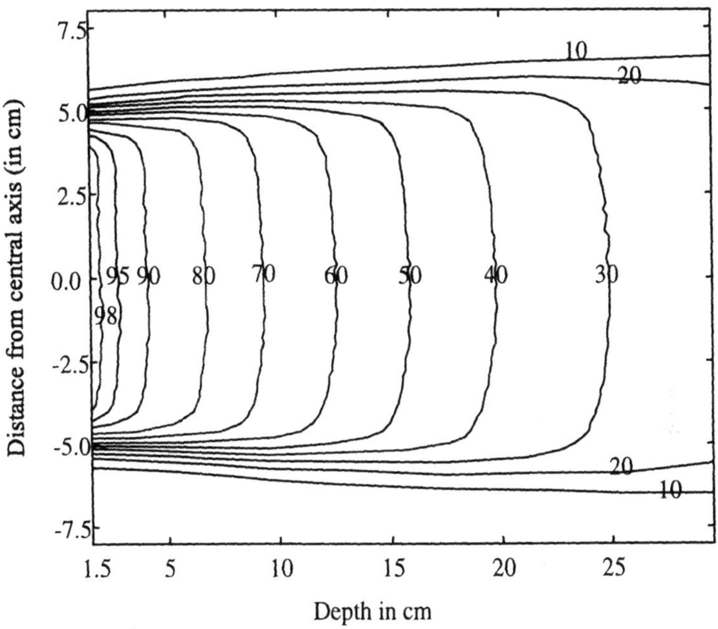

Fig. 2.10 Isodose contour plot (%DD) for a 6 MV beam, with a 10 cm by 10 cm field size, measured in a water phantom at Walsgrave Hospital NHS Trust, Coventry

2.4.5 Influence of Inhomogeneities

The human body is mainly composed of water and, as such, it is common practice to measure and calibrate the dose delivered by each linear accelerator in an open tank of water. This then permits the use of such measurements for homogeneous media. However the human body is not strictly a homogeneous medium. For example, the lungs which have a very low relative density will attenuate primary radiation much less and will produce relatively less scatter. In contrast, attenuation through bones will be higher and there will be an increase in scattered particles. As a consequence of the relative densities, transitions between regions of different densities may give rise to electronic disequilibrium, particularly for high energy photon beams. Such disequilibrium results in the creation of a build up region especially when a low density region, such as the lungs, is followed by a high density region [3, 109, 110]. Models taking into account the electronic disequilibrium [98, 109, 110] or the poly-energetic nature of the beams [3, 4, 53] have been developed. However they require an intensive computational effort and, therefore, have not been considered in this work. A more conventional approach that makes use of equivalent path length, similar to that in [116], has been adopted, although no account is taken of the electronic disequilibrium in the transition zones between two adjacent mediums of different densities. However, the model is considered to be of sufficient accuracy to demonstrate the principle of optimising a dose distribution in the presence of inhomogeneities in the pelvic region. Indeed, in the pelvic region it is noted that the differences in medium densities are less marked than in the chest and it is assumed that for scattered radiation, the gain/loss in penetrating power balances the loss/gain in the scattered radiation produced. In addition, with the amount of scattered dose being small in comparison to the primary dose contribution, the influence of inhomogeneity is modelled only via a modification of the primary attenuation. Assuming that each medium can be characterised by a linear attenuation coefficient μ_i, the dose $d(x)$ at a point of depth where $x>x_{max}$ along a given straight line path passing through k different media of respective length x_i (see Fig. 2.11) may be expressed as follows

$$d(x) = d(x_{max})\prod_{i=1}^{k} exp(-\mu_i x_i) \tag{2.4}$$

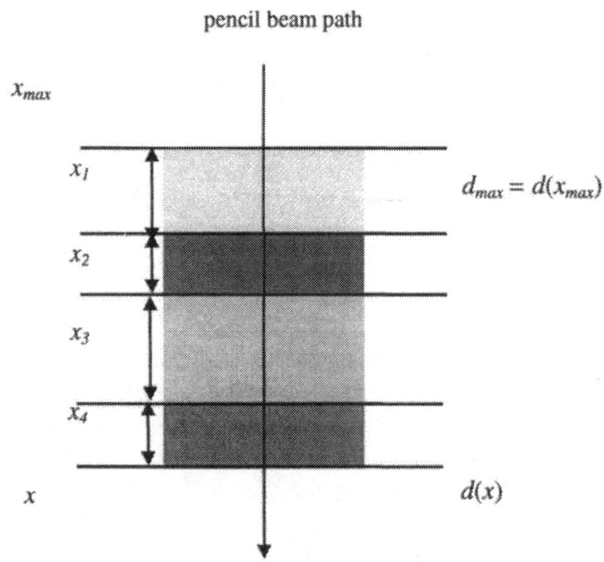

Fig. 2.11 Pencil beam path through media of different densities

Assuming that all interactions are Compton then the linear attenuation coefficients are approximately proportional to the electron densities of the various media. It is shown in [114] that electron densities with respect to water, when normalised to 1.0 (which is approximately the same as muscle), for lung and bone are approximately 0.5 and 1.5 respectively. To achieve the ratios of 0.5, 1.0 and 1.5, for lung, muscle and bone, whilst at the same time matching the CAX %DD for a 6 MV beam for normal tissue, the attenuation coefficients μ_i of equation (2.4) are taken to be $\mu_1 = 0.06$ cm^{-1}, $\mu_2 = 0.09$ cm^{-1} and $\mu_3 = 0.03$ cm^{-1}, for muscle, bone and lung respectively. It may be observed in [1] that the ratios increase only slightly for higher beam energies. In Chapter 5, where a 25 MV beam is used, the ratio between normal tissue and bone is 1.6, with the linear attenuation coefficients being $\mu_1 = 0.056$ cm^{-1} and $\mu_2 = 0.09$ cm^{-1} respectively.

Fig. 2.12 illustrates the CAX %DD depth dose for a 6 MV beam in a homogeneous medium having attenuation coefficient μ_1 (curve A) and an inhomogeneous medium (curve B). The inhomogeneous region simulated is composed of three different media with linear attenuation coefficients $\mu_1 = 0.06$ cm^{-1}, $\mu_2 = 0.09$ cm^{-1} and $\mu_3 = 0.03$ cm^{-1}, replicating muscle, bone and lung respectively.

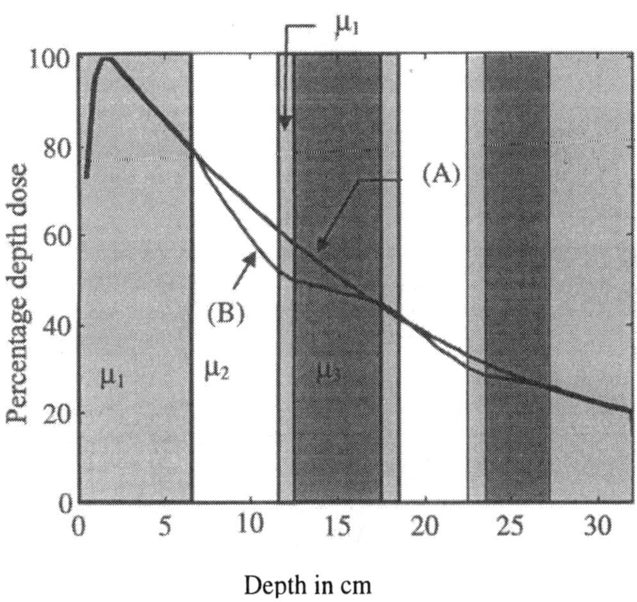

Fig. 2.12 Comparison between the CAX %DD curves for a 6 MV photon beam for a homogeneous medium (curve A) and an inhomogeneous medium (curve B)

2.5 Concept of Primary Modelling and Scatter Phenomenon

The primary component of the photon beam is modelled as a mathematical abstraction that cannot actually be measured. It can be considered as the 'ideal' component of a photon beam that is composed of uncharged ionising radiation, where the photons are assumed to lose their energy exponentially without producing scattered radiation or secondary particles [53].

The model developed separates the dose delivered by a given beam into primary and scatter contributions. The primary dose depends only on the depth for a homogeneous medium and can be computed using density weighted path lengths or equivalent path lengths for an inhomogeneous medium [53, 114]. The scatter contribution attempts to account mainly for the Compton scattering effect due to the incoming photons interacting with the body structures. Inhomogeneities can also be accounted for in the behaviour of the scattered photons in media of different densities.

Although the concept of dividing the dose into a primary and a scatter component has been criticised [110], it is still nowadays a method widely used [106, 110]. The origin of this method may be traced back to the work developed by Cunningham [59] dividing the dose into the tissue-air-ratio (TAR), that can be thought as the primary component, and the scatter-air-ratio (SAR) [116], which is a scatter function that depends on depth and field size [3, 4, 53].

2.5.1 Primary Component

The primary dose accounts for an exponentially decreasing contribution to the total dose on the central axis (the total dose is the primary dose plus that due to scatter). The scattered radiation due to interaction with human tissues increases with depth, and the amount for which the primary contribution is responsible within the total dose decreases with depth. For example at a depth of a few centimetre the primary radiation may account for as much as 95% of the total dose, whereas at depth $x \geq 10$ cm the scattered radiation may account for up to 15-20% of the total dose; with the contribution from the primary at such depths being reduced. Assuming that the measured dose comprises contributions to both primary and scatter, measured CAX %DD is modified to take into account an assumed scatter. This modified data is then used to deduce an expression for the primary dose.

The CAX %DD of the primary component (denoted $p(x)$) decreases exponentially with depth due to the photon beam attenuation as photons interact with human tissue (i.e. water). When the body structure is assumed to be homogeneous, the linear attenuation coefficient is constant (for a particular beam power) and close to the value measured in water (noting that more than 80% of the human body is composed of water [53]).

For each pencil beam $p(x)$ can thus be expressed as:
Build up region: i.e. where depth $x < x_{max}$

$$p(x) = \mathrm{cax}(x) - c_1\,(x - x_{max})^{c_2} \tag{2.5a}$$

Exponential decay region: i.e. where depth $x \geq x_{max}$

$$p(x) = x_{max}\, e^{(-c_3(x - x_{max})))} - c_4\, x + c_5\, x^2 + c_6 \tag{2.5b}$$

with the coefficients $c_i \in \Re$, i=1,...4, given in Tables 2.10 and 2.11, being obtained experimentally from the modified data with use being made of the simplex method.

Table 2.10 Coefficients describing the primary dose for a 6 MV photon beam

c_1	c_2	c_3	c_4	c_5	c_6
1.0	2.0	1.3	2.1e-2	1.8e-1	4.5e-2

Table 2.11 Coefficients describing the primary dose for a 25 MV photon beam

c_1	c_2	c_3	c_4	c_5	c_6
1.0e-1	1.0	5.6e-2	9.0e-2	0.0	0.0

Figures 2.13 and 2.14 illustrate the breakdown that is obtained, when the total dose is decomposed in terms of the primary and scatter contributions for 6 MV and 25 MV photon beams. The dashed lines shows the primary, obtained respectively from equations 2.5a and 2.5b, and the solid lines shows the total dose measured. The deficit between the measured dose and the modelled primary dose is assumed to be the contribution due to scatter.

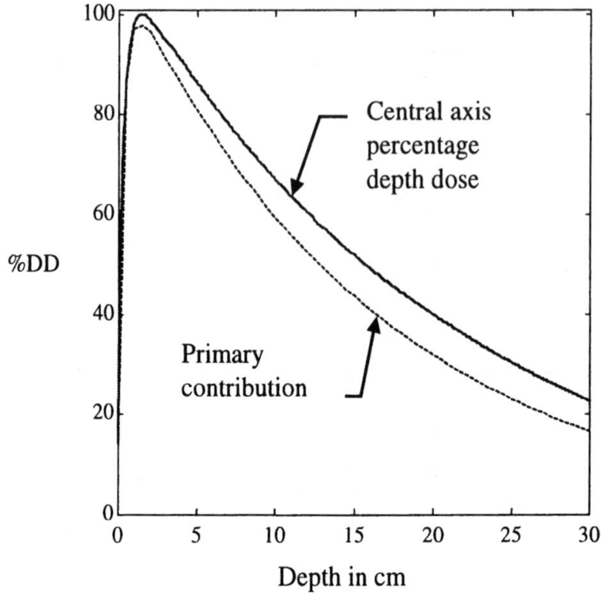

Fig. 2.13 Primary compared to central axis central percentage depth dose for a 6 MV beam

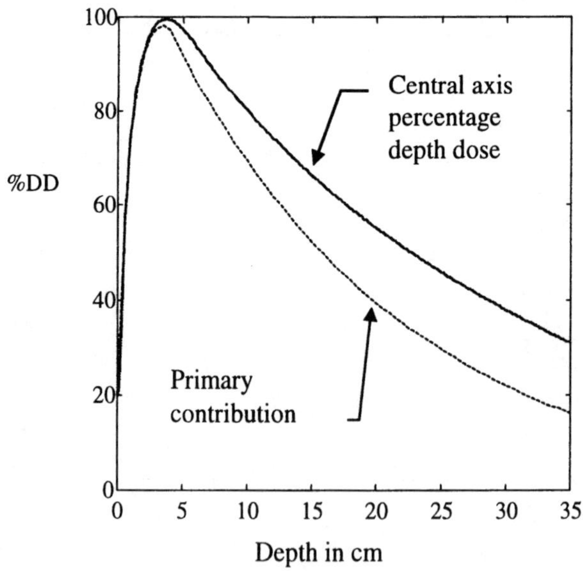

Fig. 2.14 Primary compared to central axis central percentage depth dose for a 25 MV beam

The resulting isodose plot with the beam assumed to be composed of primary radiation only would be 'flat'. In practice, however, isodose contours of X-ray photon beams are non flat due to the physical characteristics of the linacs and the physical interactions between the beam radiation and the human body.

2.5.2 Forward Scatter Phenomenon

An analogy to the physical nature of the scatter can be drawn if all the small scatter contributions are thought of as the small interactions that take place between scattered electrons and photons with matter. In this work, it is convenient to consider the interaction of the individual pencil beams with matter. Essentially it is assumed that the individual pencil beams interact with matter at discrete depths, depositing their energy to elemental cells belonging to a Cartesian matrix grid. (For an individual beam this is termed a beam dose matrix, see Chap. 3.) An illustration of such concept is given in Fig. 2.15, which shows the intersection of *n* notional pencil beams with *m* discrete depths into the body tissues. In this way, it is assumed that all grid points from depth 0 to *j*-1 contribute to the scattered radiation received by grid points at depth *j* (see Fig. 2.15). Consequently the scattered dose d_{Sij} received at a grid point (*i,j*) may be expressed as:

$$d_{Sij} = \sum_{i=1}^{n} \sum_{k=1}^{j-1} f_s(i,k) \tag{2.6}$$

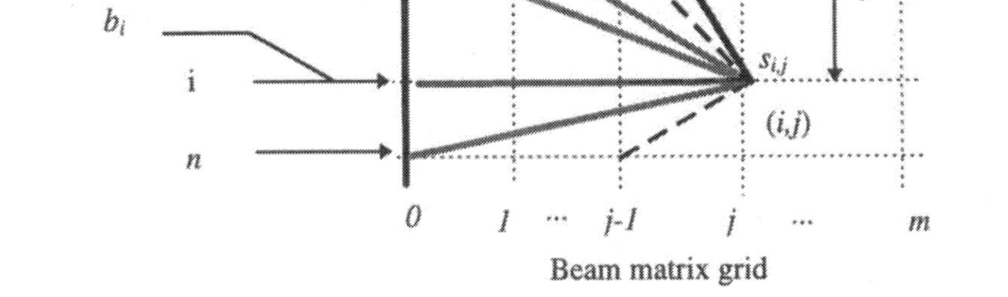

Fig. 2.15 Sum of elemental scatter contributions to a point (*i,j*) on the beam matrix grid

The introduction of a scatter component enables a model to replicate the dose on the edges of the beam and the interactions between the individual pencil beams that compose the overall beam. The scatter in the model is aimed to reproduce the increase of the dose at the centre of the field with respect to the dose on each side of the central axis. The scatter process modelled in this work, attempts to approximate the overall process of diffusion of scattered radiation and assumes that the energy scattered is transferred in forward and sideways directions only, with the backscatter effect and the scatter outside the beam path assumed to be negligible.

At the elemental cell level, each scatter contribution can be considered as being a variable amount of primary radiation transmitted from cell to cell mainly in the forward direction but also on the side. In an attempt to replicate the effects of the interaction between photons and electrons with matter, i.e. mainly Compton interaction, a relationship is to be derived to replicate the effects observed. The elemental scatter contribution may be expressed as a function of the angle of the incoming scattering radiation, the distance between the elemental cells emitting the scattered radiation and the elemental cells collecting or receiving it, see Fig. 2.15. With reference to Fig. 2.15, it can be shown that the scatter contribution at a given point in the beam dose matrix may be approximated by the expression:

$$d_{Sij} = \sum_{i=1}^{n} \sum_{k=1}^{j-1} \frac{e^{-\sigma(r\sin(\theta))^2}}{r} \tag{2.7}$$

where r is the distance between the source of the emitted scattered radiation and the collecting matrix grid point considered and θ is the angle between the central axis and the lines connecting the emitting source points to the point considered. For both parallel and divergent beams r^2 and θ are given respectively by: $r^2 = \delta i^2 + \delta j^2$ and $\theta = sin^{-1}\ (\delta i\ /\ r)$, see Chap. 3. The scalar σ, related to the attenuation coefficient, is determined empirically in the following section.

2.5.3 Determination of the Coefficient σ

The scatter contribution is maximum for ($\theta = 0$) which occurs when the points interacting lie along the same pencil beam. The higher the value of θ, the lower the scatter contribution. The scattered dose on the beam CAX is fixed since it is deduced from the primary dose level on the CAX (see Chap. 3). The beam curvature is a function of the scalar σ, where an increase in σ results in a reduction of the dose on each side of the beam CAX, thus increasing the beam curvature. Figures 2.16 and 2.17 show, respectively, (i) the effect of scatter from a point source on the CAX and (ii) the overall scatter contribution due to 25 equispaced equally weighted pencil beams.

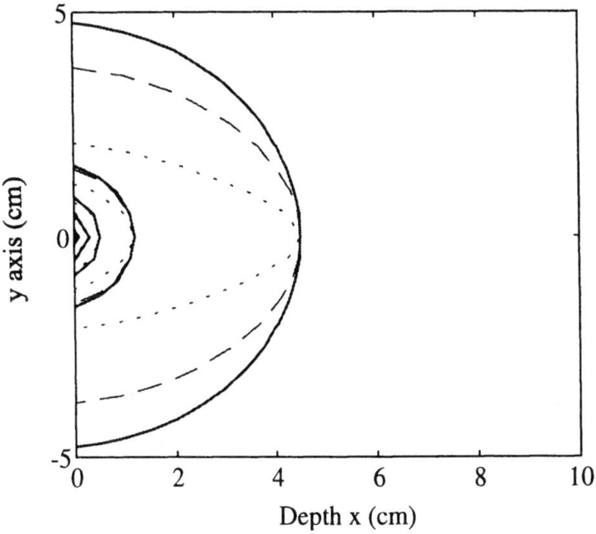

Fig. 2.16 Variation in the normalised elemental scatter contribution from a point source with $\sigma = 0.002$ represented by the solid lines, $\sigma = 0.02$ represented by the dashed lines and $\sigma = 0.2$ represented by the dotted lines

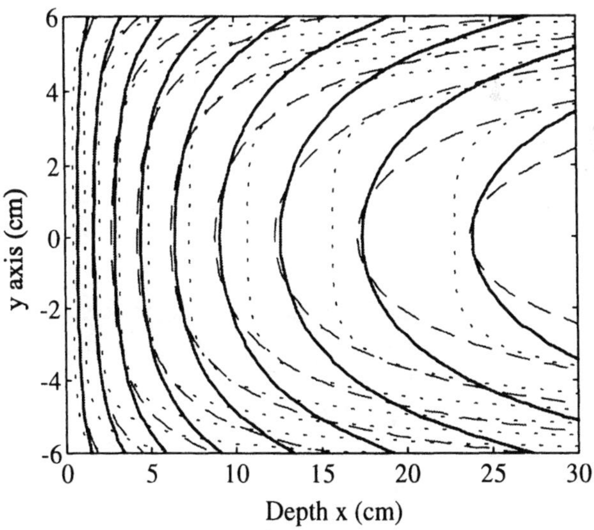

Fig. 2.17 Variation in the overall scatter contribution from 25 equispaced equally weighted pencil beams, with $\sigma = 0.002$ represented by the solid lines, $\sigma = 0.02$ represented by the dashed lines and $\sigma = 0.2$ represented by the dotted lines

In order to obtain a value for the scalar σ, it is convenient to formulate a measure of the resulting match between measured and calculated data. In this context, the value of σ is found by minimising the mean value of the absolute error between measured and calculated data for a range of typical beam profiles. Here use is made of an open field beam as well as three intensity modulated beams. For each beam an overall % mean error value $\bar{e}$ is defined as:

$$\bar{e} = \frac{\sum_{i=1}^{n}\sum_{j=1}^{m} e_{ij}\%}{mn} \tag{2.8}$$

where the subscripts ij denote the elements of the $n\times m$ beam dose matrix and $e_{ij}\%$ corresponds to the absolute error expressed as a percentage between actual measured and calculated doses, i.e.

$$\{e_{ij}\%\} = \left\{\left(\frac{|d_a - d_c|}{d_a}\right)_{ij} \times 100\right\} \tag{2.9}$$

where d_a and d_c denote the actual measured and calculated doses at the $n\times m$ points in the dose matrix grid considered.

When considering the overall aggregate of the % mean errors arising from the use of a fixed value of σ for N_{Beam} beams, an overall aggregate value of the % mean error is given by

$$\tilde{e} = \sum_{k=1}^{N_{Beam}} \bar{e}_k \Big/ N_{Beam} \tag{2.10}$$

is adopted; with the most appropriate value of σ being that which minimises $\tilde{e}$. In this work the value of σ which has been obtained empirically, as outlined above, for a 6 MV beam is found to be $\sigma = 2.0e^{-2}$. This gives rise to a mean error, in terms of percentage, for an open field of 1.57% (i.e. <1.6%) and an overall mean error, in terms of percentage, for an open field and three intensity modulated fields of 1.95% (i.e. < 2.0%), see Table 2.12. This level of error is considered to be acceptable from an experimental modelling view point.

Table 2.12 Influence of σ on the percentage mean of absolute error $\overline{e}$ for four different beam profiles and on the overall aggregate percentage mean absolute error $\widetilde{e}$ between measured and calculated data for a 10 cm by 10 cm 6 MV beam

Beam profile		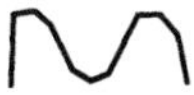	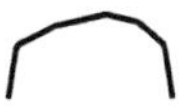	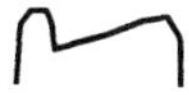	Aggregate % mean error $\widetilde{e}$
σ	% mean error $\overline{e}$				
$1.5e^{-2}$	1.563	2.556	1.855	1.827	1.948
$1.75e^{-2}$	1.565	2.548	1.858	1.819	1.947
$1.1975e^{-2}$	1.569	2.544	1.865	1.807	1.946
$2.0e^{-2}$	1.570	2.543	1.867	1.805	1.946
$2.203e^{-2}$	1.571	2.542	1.868	1.804	1.946
$2.5e^{-2}$	1.61	2.517	1.920	1.779	1.955

The elemental variation of scatter, as a function of both scattering angle and the distance from the source of the emitting scatter, when $\sigma = 2.0e^{-2}$, is shown in Fig. 2.18. The scatter contribution decays exponentially as the radius increases. The back-scatter effect being assumed to be negligible for the beam considered; the scatter source contributes only in the forward and sideways directions.

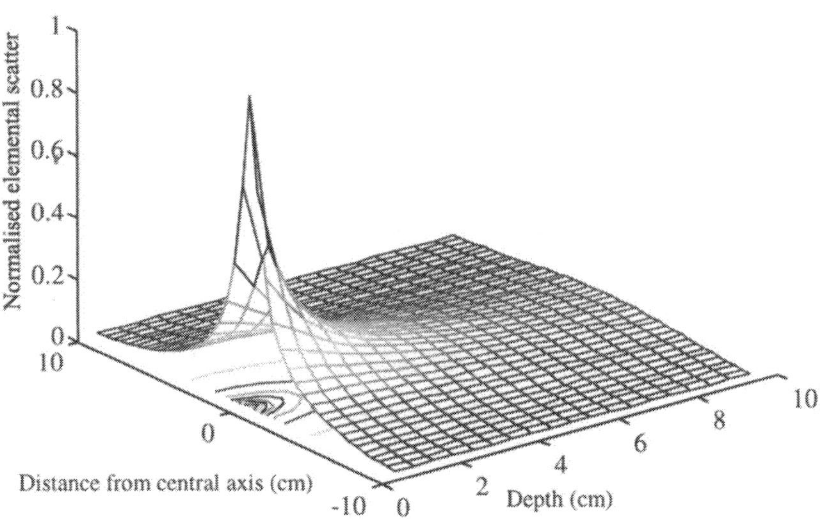

Fig. 2.18 Normalised scatter contribution originating from a single matrix element given in terms of depth and distance from the point of emission situated on the central axis

2.6 Concluding Remarks

This Chapter has introduced the basic features which characterise a photon beam and has highlighted the need for a model which adequately replicates the relevant physical phenomena. The model developed is used (in Chap. 4) for the purpose of calculating the optimum set of intensity modulated beams (individual pencil beams) to accurately achieve some desired dose distribution.

In order to provide an appreciation of the physical characteristics of a photon beam, terms such as, central axis (CAX), central axis percentage depth dose (CAX %DD), in-air-profile (IAP), penumbra and the effect of inhomogeneities have been introduced and discussed.

Fundamental to much of the work that is presented in this work is the concept of primary and scattered radiation. Indeed it is the inclusion of these two contributions that is very much central to the matrix based beam model developed in Chap. 3. The necessary assumptions made and the preliminary steps towards the formulation of a matrix based model have been introduced.

CHAPTER 3

FORMULATION OF MATRIX BASED BEAM MODEL

3.1 Introduction

Having highlighted in Chap. 2 the fundamental underlying physical characteristics of a photon beam, this Chap. develops a matrix based beam model which is used for the purpose of optimisation of the intensity modulated beams (or individual pencil beams). Essentially the inputs to the model (which are required to be optimised) are the resulting intensity modulated beam (IMB) profiles of a predetermined number of beams in a given treatment plan. (It is shown later in Chap. 5 that it is also possible to optimise the number and orientation of the beams prior to optimising their IMBs.)

By first considering parallel pencil beams, Chap. 3 develops the matrix formulation of a beam model. Whilst in reality the beams are divergent, the parallel pencil beam model is shown in Chap. 4 to provide an effective tool for obtaining near optimal solutions prior to fine tuning using a divergent beam model. Building on the special case of the parallel beam, the model is extended to accommodate for the case of a divergent beam. A number of different ways of exploiting both parallel and divergent beam models are discussed.

The parallel beam formulation lends itself well to the solution of the inverse problem using techniques of iterative least squares, see Chap. 4, whilst the divergent beam lends itself to forward solving methods such as genetic algorithms, see Chap. 5. Hybrid methods which combine the parallel and divergent approaches are discussed in Chap. 6.

The aim of the matrix formulation of the beam model is to provide a relationship between the IMBs, which can be considered as the inputs to the system, and the dose distribution resulting from a particular set of IMBs, which can be considered as the output of the system. As such, each beam is regarded as a sub system that is defined by the type of beam used (here 6 MV and 25 MV photon beams are considered), the geometry of the patient and the shape of the internal ROIs and their respective inhomogeneities. The matrix formulation reflects the fact that the dose at any given point is considered to be the sum of a primary component and a scatter component. The formulation of the primary dose calculation matrix, including inhomogeneity and patient contour correction, is considered first. Attention is then focused on the formulation of the scatter dose calculation matrix that can be added to the primary dose calculation matrix to form the overall beam dose calculation matrix. The resulting beam dose calculation matrix expresses the dose at any given point in the dose calculation grid as a function of all the IMBs composing the particular beam described.

The model developed separates the dose delivered by a given beam into primary and scatter contributions. The primary dose depends only on the depth for a homogeneous medium and can be computed using density weighted path lengths or equivalent path lengths for an inhomogeneous medium [53, 109, 116]. The scatter contribution attempts to account mainly for the Compton scattering effect due to the incoming photons interacting with the body structures. Inhomogeneities can also be accounted for in the behaviour of the scattered photons in media of different densities.

3.2 Parallel Pencil Beam Model Formulation

3.2.1 The Parallel Matrix Grid

In this work a 2-D pencil beam model expressed in matrix form is developed. A pencil beam formulation assumes that each beam involved in a treatment plan can be decomposed into elemental pencil beams. The intensity of each of these pencil beams can be modified independently by the optimisation algorithm to produce an intensity modulated beam (IMB) [108]. Elemental pencil beams are taken as being synonymous with IMBs and the intensity modulation is realised by means of patient specific compensators. Attenuation of each pencil beam is realised as a function of the thickness (or height) of the compensating material inserted into the pencil beam path (see Chap. 6). The aim of the matrix formulation is to predict the 2-D dose distribution resulting from a beam profile that corresponds to the intensities associated with each of the pencil beams.

For the purpose of illustration, and to assist with the formulation of the beam model, a single beam is initially considered. The beam is assumed to enter the patient from the left side (see Fig. 3.1). The treatment region is represented as a 2-D treatment grid that corresponds to a computed tomography (CT) slice. Without loss of generality, consideration is given to the rectangular shaped N by M reference grid onto which each elemental beam is superimposed, see Fig. 3.1.

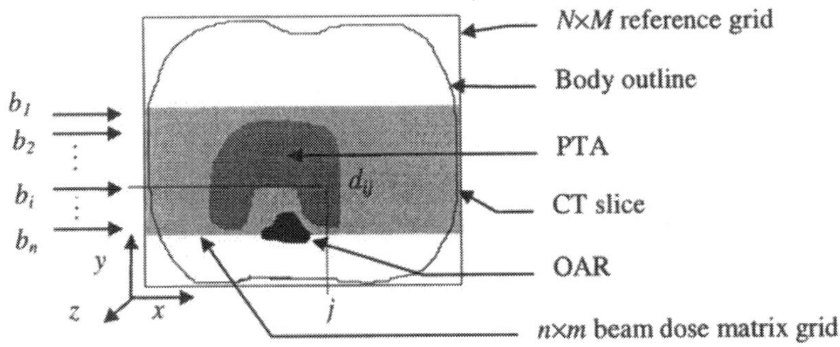

Fig. 3.1 Parallel beam dose matrix in the $N \times M$ reference grid

The elements within the columns of the beam dose matrix correspond to depth dose whilst the elements within the rows represent the dose along the pencil beam paths. Each point within the beam dose matrix corresponds to the notional intersection of a pencil beam with lines orthogonal to the central axis and separated by a distance (depth) $\Delta x = 0.5$ cm, where each column corresponds to a particular depth. The first column corresponds to the beam entry point closest to the beam source, whereas the last column corresponds to the beam exit point further away from the source. Each row represents the path of a pencil beam. Each pencil beam is separated by a distance Δy. For parallel pencil beams this distance remains the same (see Fig. 3.2), whereas for divergent pencil beams Δy increases with depth.

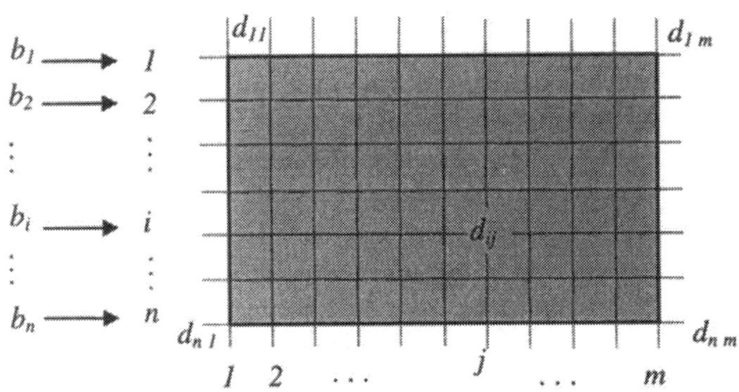

Fig. 3.2 Grid representing the parallel beam dose matrix

Given the location of the cancerous region considered in this work (i.e. the pelvic region) together with the spatial resolution that can be obtained from the patient specific compensators developed (see Chap. 6), Δy = 0.5 cm is considered to give a good compromise between speed of calculation and accuracy of the solution which is physically achievable. (However, for head and neck treatment and small cancerous regions, a finer resolution may be required.) The number of IMBs per beam is calculated such that all the PTA is irradiated, and is given by the following expression:

$$n = roundup(\text{FS} / \Delta y) \tag{3.1}$$

where the field size (FS) is given by the projection of the PTA onto the patient surface, Δy is the distance separating two neighbouring IMBs at the skin level and *roundup* is defined such that FS/Δy is rounded up to the next integer value.

3.2.2 Beam Dose Matrix

Consider the $N\times M$ reference grid which encompasses the patient cross sectional area (i.e. the area of a CT slice), see Fig. 3.3. In the development of the beam matrix model it is convenient to superimpose the beam dose matrix directly onto the patient's reference grid.

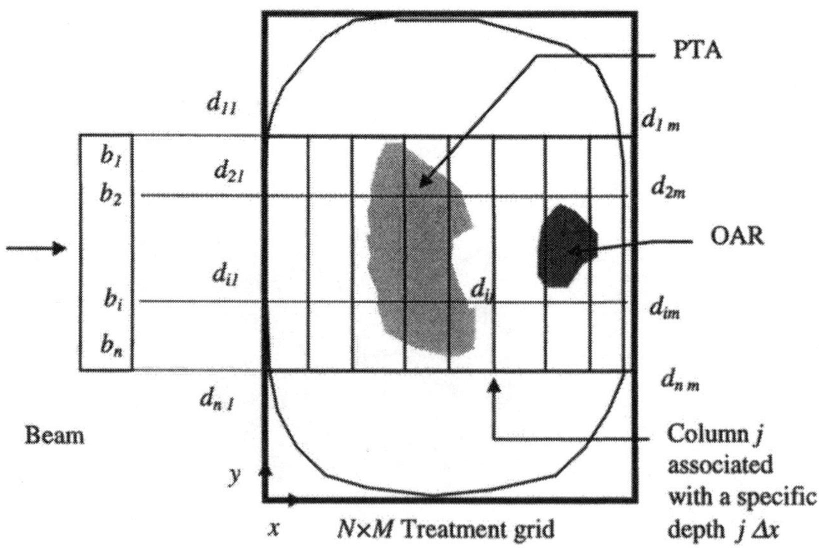

Fig. 3.3 Representation of the beam dose matrix within the overall reference grid

The beam dose matrix for an individual parallel beam, as illustrated in Fig. 3.3, may be expressed mathematically by defining the beam dose matrix $\mathbf{D} \in \Re^{n \times m}$

$$D = \{d_{ij}\} = \begin{bmatrix} d_{11} & d_{12} & \cdots & d_{1m} \\ d_{21} & d_{22} & \cdots & d_{2m} \\ \vdots & \vdots & & \vdots \\ d_{n1} & d_{n2} & \cdots & d_{nm} \end{bmatrix} \tag{3.2}$$

where each row corresponds to the dose delivered along a pencil beam, i=1...n, and each column, j=1...m, corresponds to a depth (from left to right) into the patient body. The matrix grid elements are separated by an amount Δy and Δx (between rows and columns respectively) which, for the pelvic region, are taken as $\Delta y = \Delta x = 0.5$ cm.

The dose d_{ij} delivered to each element within the beam matrix grid comprises a dose due to primary, denoted $d_{p_{ij}}$, and a dose due to scatter, denoted $d_{s_{ij}}$ so that:

$$\{d_{ij}\} = \{ d_{p_{ij}} \} + \{ d_{s_{ij}} \} \tag{3.3}$$

alternatively $\mathbf{D} = \mathbf{D}_p + \mathbf{D}_s$ (3.4)

In the development of the matrix based beam model, the primary dose $d_{p_{ij}}$ and the scatter dose $d_{s_{ij}}$ are considered separately; with the primary dose matrix $\mathbf{D}_p$ being considered first. In order to proceed it is convenient to express the beam dose matrix $\mathbf{D} \in \Re^{n \times m}$ as a partitioned vector $\mathbf{d} \in \Re^{nm}$, such that: $\mathbf{d} = \mathbf{d}_p + \mathbf{d}_s$
i.e.

$$d = \begin{bmatrix} d_{11} \\ d_{21} \\ \vdots \\ d_{n1} \\ -- \\ \vdots \\ -- \\ d_{1m} \\ d_{2m} \\ \vdots \\ d_{nm} \end{bmatrix} = \begin{bmatrix} \mathbf{d}_1 \\ -- \\ \vdots \\ -- \\ \mathbf{d}_m \end{bmatrix} = \begin{bmatrix} \mathbf{d}_{p_1} \\ -- \\ \vdots \\ -- \\ \mathbf{d}_{p_m} \end{bmatrix} + \begin{bmatrix} \mathbf{d}_{s_1} \\ -- \\ \vdots \\ -- \\ \mathbf{d}_{s_m} \end{bmatrix} \tag{3.5}$$

Attention is now focused towards the primary dose matrix and the scatter dose matrix.

3.2.3 Primary Dose Calculation Matrix

For a homogeneous medium with a flat surface and modulated beams of the same intensity, the primary component of the beam is assumed to produce an ideal dose distribution with flat isodose contours and no scatter. As a consequence all points at the same depth receive the same amount of radiation. Also, when considering the primary contribution in isolation, each IMB affects only the beam matrix grid points in the modulated pencil beam path, i.e. no lateral interaction is observed. The dose $d_{p_{ij}}$ received by the grid points located at a depth $x = j$ on the beam matrix grid and facing the ith IMB is given by

$$d_{p_{ij}} = p_{ij}\, b_i, \tag{3.6}$$

with $b_i \geq 0$ are the normalised modulated beam intensities and the p_{ij} are elements describing the primary attenuation of the beam and relate to equations (2.4), (2.5a) and (2.5b) of Chap. 2. Repeating this procedure for each elemental intensity modulated beam, $i = 1...n$, the primary dose received by the elements at depth j can be expressed in the following matrix form:

$$\begin{bmatrix} d_{p_{1j}} \\ d_{p_{2j}} \\ \vdots \\ d_{p_{nj}} \end{bmatrix} = \begin{bmatrix} p_{1j} & 0 & \cdots & 0 \\ 0 & p_{2j} & \ddots & \vdots \\ \vdots & \ddots & \ddots & 0 \\ 0 & \cdots & 0 & p_{nj} \end{bmatrix} \begin{bmatrix} b_1 \\ b_2 \\ \vdots \\ b_n \end{bmatrix} \quad \text{or} \quad \mathbf{d}_{p_j} = \mathbf{P}_j \mathbf{b} \tag{3.7}$$

Repeating this procedure for each depth $j = 1...m$, the primary dose calculation matrix can be expressed in partitioned form as follows:

$$\mathbf{P} = [\mathbf{P}_1\ \mathbf{P}_2\ ...\ \mathbf{P}_m]^{\mathrm{T}} \tag{3.8}$$

where the diagonal matrices $\mathbf{P}_j \in \Re^{n\times n}$ describe the primary dose attenuation for each successive depth of the beam dose matrix.

The primary dose contribution to the beam dose matrix is given by the following expression

$$\mathbf{d}_p = \mathbf{P}\ \mathbf{b} \tag{3.9}$$

The primary dose calculation matrix $\mathbf{P}$ is a $(n\times m)\times n$ matrix which relates to a set of $(n\times m)$ linear equations with n unknowns, where $n << m$ corresponds to the elemental intensity modulated beams (i.e. the pencil beams) that influence the dose at $(n\times m)$ points in the beam dose matrix. It should be noted that the primary dose calculation matrix is a sparse matrix, and this can be exploited to advantage since it reduces the amount of storage required.

3.2.4 Scatter Dose Calculation Matrix

The scatter formulation in matrix form aims to replicate the increase in scattered radiation with depth, with respect to the initial incoming photons. As the photon penetrates deeper into the body, scattered photons and electrons are created [53] and these themselves become the source of new scattered radiation. As the photons undergo atomic reactions, they lose some of their energy and penetrating power. As a consequence the closer the source of scattered radiation, the higher the resulting scatter contribution [53].

With the scatter being assumed to be a forward process, the total scatter received by the jth depth in the beam dose matrix is the sum of all the scatter emanating from the preceding layers up to the point of beam entry. For example, the scattered dose received by a point located on the ith pencil beam, and j^{th} depth, is composed of scatter emanating from all elements on the second, third ... up to and including the $(j\text{-}1)^{th}$ depth; the lowest attenuation being associated with the scatter emitted from the elements corresponding to the $(j\text{-}1)^{th}$ depth on the same pencil beam, i.e. the $i(j\text{-}1)$ element. The only exception is the first layer of elemental cells which have no preceding layers emitting scattered radiation. It is assumed that the dose received by the first layer is only due to the primary. Similarly, the dose in the build up region is assumed to be composed mainly of a primary component, with only a small portion of the dose due to scatter. This assumption may appear to be over simplistic, but the reason for its choice is that it simplifies the scatter model and yet still provides an acceptable model of the beam characteristics in the region close to the skin. Indeed, the developed approach compares favourably to other models developed previously for optimisation purposes that do not consider the dose in the build up region; and only focuses on modelling the exponential decay region [36, 37, 100, 103].

Making use of the above assumptions, two different approaches have been considered to model the effect of radiation in the body structures. The first approach, which was later superseded, considered the scattered dose as a quantity linked to the primary dose, whereas in the second approach the scatter is modelled independently to the primary.

Initial Formulation. In the initial formulation it was assumed that the scatter contribution depended only on the primary dose received; with the scatter being a secondary effect [106, 107, 108]. By considering the dose delivered as a two stage process, each cell receives a primary dose and an additional dose due to scatter. Figure 3.4 represents scattered interaction between cells located on the $(j\text{-}k)^{th}$ depth (or column) emitting scattered radiation towards a receiving cell located on the jth column of the beam matrix grid.

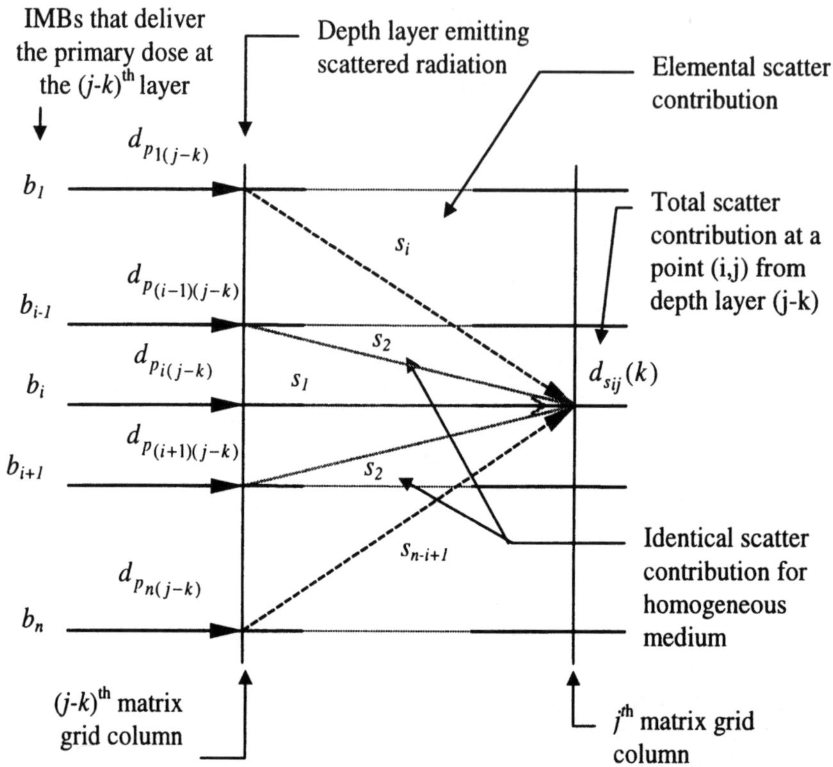

Fig. 3.4 Scatter contribution to a point (i,j) incoming from the n elements of the $(j\text{-}k)^{th}$ matrix grid column

In general, the scattered dose received at a point (i,j) in the ith pencil beam on the jth column from the $(j\text{-}k)^{th}$ depth layer can be expressed as follows:

$$d_{s_{ij}}(j|j\text{-}k) = s_i(j|j\text{-}k)\, d_{p_{1(j-k)}} + \ldots + s_2(j|\,j\text{-}k)\, d_{p_{(i-1)(j-k)}} + s_1(j|\,j\text{-}k)\ d_{p_{i(j-k)}} + \ldots$$
$$\ldots + s_2(j|\,j\text{-}k)\ d_{p_{(i+1)(j-k)}} + s_{n-i+1}(j|\,j\text{-}k)\ d_{p_{n(j-k)}} \tag{3.10}$$

i.e.

$$d_{s_{ij}}(j|j\text{-}k) = \sum_{h=1}^{n} s_{|h-i+1|}(j\,|\,j-k)\, d_{p(|h-i+1|,\,j-k)} \tag{3.11}$$

where the notation $(j|j\text{-}k)$ defines the scatter from the $(j\text{-}k)^{th}$ layer to the jth layer. Note that the notation $|h-i+1|$ which corresponds to the absolute value of the index $h\text{-}i\text{+}1$ is used to indicate that the scattered contributions are assumed to be symmetrical with respect to the ith pencil beam (in the case of a flat patient contour and homogeneous medium).

Repeating this process for each point of the jth column receiving scatter from the $(j-k)^{th}$ column, and expressing the resulting set of equations into a matrix form gives:

$$\begin{bmatrix} d_{s1j} \\ d_{s2j} \\ \vdots \\ d_{snj} \end{bmatrix}_{(j|j-k)} = \begin{bmatrix} s_1 & s_2 & \cdots & s_n \\ s_2 & s_1 & \cdots & s_{n-1} \\ \vdots & & \ddots & \vdots \\ s_n & \cdots & s_2 & s_1 \end{bmatrix}_{j-k} \begin{bmatrix} d_{p1(j-k)} \\ d_{p2(j-k)} \\ \vdots \\ d_{pn(j-k)} \end{bmatrix} \tag{3.12}$$

i.e.

$$\mathbf{d}_{sj}(j \mid j-k) = \mathbf{S}_{j-k}\mathbf{d}_{p(j-k)} \tag{3.13}$$

The total scatter received by all the elemental cells at a given depth (i.e. columns having smaller indices than the one considered) is the sum of all the scatter emitted by each point in the path of the pencil beams from the point of beam entry to the layer considered:

$$\mathbf{d}_{sj} = \sum_{i=1}^{j} \mathbf{S}_i \mathbf{d}_{pj-i+1} \tag{3.14}$$

This can be expressed into the following partitioned matrix form:

$$\mathbf{d}_{sj} = \begin{bmatrix} \mathbf{S}_j & \mathbf{S}_{j-1} & \cdots & \mathbf{S}_1 \end{bmatrix} \begin{bmatrix} \mathbf{d}_{p1} \\ \mathbf{d}_{p2} \\ \vdots \\ \mathbf{d}_{pj} \end{bmatrix} \tag{3.15}$$

where $\mathbf{S}_i$, $i = 2...j$, are scatter matrices describing the scatter contribution from the previous layers, noting that $\mathbf{S}_1=\mathbf{0}$, due to the fact that scatter is emitted only from previous layers and not from the layer considered.

Assuming a grid representing a parallel beam dose matrix, with equal spacing between rows and columns across the beam, and provided that each elemental scatter contribution is obtained from equation (2.7), then the matrix $\mathbf{S}_i$ describing the scatter attenuation between two depth layers separated in depth by i-1 layers is constant. Indeed, equation (2.7) ensures that the attenuation depends only on the relative location of the points emitting the scatter with respect to the points receiving the scatter. Making use of the above assumptions, the following matrix expression relating the partitioned scatter contributions in terms of the primary contributions can then be deduced

$$\begin{bmatrix} \mathbf{d}_{s_1} \\ \mathbf{d}_{s_2} \\ \mathbf{d}_{s_3} \\ \vdots \\ \mathbf{d}_{s_m} \end{bmatrix} = \begin{bmatrix} \mathbf{S}_1 & \mathbf{0} & \mathbf{0} & \cdots & \mathbf{0} \\ \mathbf{S}_2 & \mathbf{S}_1 & \mathbf{0} & \cdots & \mathbf{0} \\ \mathbf{S}_3 & \mathbf{S}_2 & \mathbf{S}_1 & \mathbf{0} & \mathbf{0} \\ \vdots & \ddots & \ddots & \ddots & \vdots \\ \mathbf{S}_m & \cdots & \mathbf{S}_3 & \mathbf{S}_2 & \mathbf{S}_1 \end{bmatrix} \begin{bmatrix} \mathbf{d}_{p_1} \\ \mathbf{d}_{p_2} \\ \mathbf{d}_{p_3} \\ \vdots \\ \mathbf{d}_{p_m} \end{bmatrix} \tag{3.16}$$

or

$$\mathbf{d}_s = \mathbf{S}\,\mathbf{d}_p \tag{3.17}$$

where $\mathbf{d}_p$ is the primary dose vector, $\mathbf{d}_s$ is the scattered dose vector, and $\mathbf{S}$ is the lower triangular block partitioned beam scatter calculation matrix. Note that the matrix $\mathbf{S}$ can be interpreted as follows:

The closer to the beam entry point to the depth layer receiving scatter, the less likely it is to receive a large amount of scatter. The deeper into the body, the more likely is the dose to be a combination of multiple scattering. With $\mathbf{S}_1 = \mathbf{0}$, the first layer of cells does not receive any scatter. At depth m, the layer receives scatter from all the preceding layers.

From (3.17) it may be deduced that since:

$$\mathbf{d} = \mathbf{d}_p + \mathbf{d}_s \tag{3.18}$$

then

$$\mathbf{d} = \mathbf{d}_p + \mathbf{S}\mathbf{d}_p \tag{3.19}$$

and from (3.9) it follows that

$$\mathbf{d} = [\mathbf{P}+\mathbf{SP}]\mathbf{b} \tag{3.20}$$

The above approach is used in [106, 108] and the resulting doses were compared with CAX data given in Supplement 17 of the BJR for 6 MV and 10 MV beams [25]. In order to match the reference data, it was necessary to re-scale the amount of scatter delivered to each depth. The reason for this is that the initial approach to modelling the scatter tends to produce a scatter component that ‘follows’ the primary, i.e. increases exponentially in the build up region and then decreases exponentially as the primary decays with depth.

Whilst, the initial approach provided and insight into the beam model formulation it was subsequently superseded in favour of a modified formulation. In the modified formulation, the scatter is modelled independently from the primary. This removes the need to re-scale the amount of scatter for each depth, and only requires the scaling of the scatter at a reference point to account for changes in field size. This has obvious practical advantages.

Modified Formulation. In the modified approach, the scatter is considered as an independent function to the primary component of the dose, whilst depending on the intensity of the individual pencil beams. Adopting the same notation as in the initial approach, the scatter at a point (i,j) is given by

$$d_{s_{ij}}(j|j\text{-}k) = s_i(j|\,j\text{-}k)b_1 + ... + s_2(j|\,j\text{-}k)b_{i-1} + s_1(j|\,j\text{-}k)b_i + s_2(j|\,j\text{-}k)b_{i+1} + ... + s_{n-i+1}(j|\,j\text{-}k)b_n \tag{3.21}$$

Making use of the same principle, the matrix formulation of the scattered dose received from a layer at a distance k columns becomes*:

$$\begin{bmatrix} d_{s_{1j}} \\ d_{s_{2j}} \\ \vdots \\ d_{s_{nj}} \end{bmatrix}_{(j|j-k)} = \begin{bmatrix} s_1 & s_2 & \cdots & s_n \\ s_2 & s_1 & \cdots & s_{n-1} \\ \vdots & & \ddots & \vdots \\ s_n & \cdots & s_2 & s_1 \end{bmatrix}_{j-k} \begin{bmatrix} 1 & 0 & \cdots & 0 \\ 0 & 1 & & \\ \vdots & & \ddots & \\ 0 & & & 1 \end{bmatrix} \begin{bmatrix} b_1 \\ b_2 \\ \vdots \\ b_n \end{bmatrix} \tag{3.22}$$

$$\mathbf{d}_{s_j}(j\,|\,j-k) = \mathbf{S}_{j\text{-}k}\mathbf{Ib} \tag{3.23}$$

where the primary dose vector of (3.13) is effectively replaced by the identity matrix multiplied by the IMB vector **b**.

Note that the components of the elemental scatter matrices are given by

$$s = \frac{e^{-\sigma(r\sin(\theta))^2}}{r} \tag{3.24}$$

where, with reference to Fig. 3.4, r is the distance between the source of the scatter radiation and the point considered, θ is the angle between the central axis and a line joining the source points to the point considered and σ is a coefficient found empirically, see Chap. 2. For both parallel and divergent beams r^2 and θ are given respectively by:

$$r^2 = (a\Delta y)^2 + (b\Delta x)^2 \text{ and } \theta = sin^{-1}(a\Delta y\,/\,r) \tag{3.25}$$

where a and b are integer multiples of the elemental cells separating the source and the recipient points of scatter.

It follows that $s_1 > s_2 > ... > s_n$ where s_1 represents the highest scatter contribution emanating from a cell lying on the same pencil beam as the cell (or point) receiving the scatter.

---

* Note that whilst the identity matrix is not necessary for the above expression, it becomes useful when dealing with the overall scatter formulation.

$$\begin{bmatrix} d_{s_{1j}} \\ d_{s_{2j}} \\ \vdots \\ d_{s_{nj}} \end{bmatrix} = \left[\begin{bmatrix} s_1 & s_2 & \cdots & s_n \\ s_2 & s_1 & \cdots & s_{n-1} \\ \vdots & & \ddots & \vdots \\ s_n & \cdots & s_2 & s_1 \end{bmatrix}_j \cdots \begin{bmatrix} s_1 & s_2 & \cdots & s_n \\ s_2 & s_1 & \cdots & s_{n-1} \\ \vdots & & \ddots & \vdots \\ s_n & \cdots & s_2 & s_1 \end{bmatrix}_1 \right] \begin{bmatrix} \begin{bmatrix} 1 & 0 & \cdots & 0 \\ 0 & 1 & & \\ \vdots & & \ddots & \\ 0 & & & 1 \end{bmatrix}_1 \\ \vdots \\ \begin{bmatrix} 1 & 0 & \cdots & 0 \\ 0 & 1 & & \\ \vdots & & \ddots & \\ 0 & & & 1 \end{bmatrix}_j \end{bmatrix} \begin{bmatrix} b_1 \\ b_2 \\ \vdots \\ b_n \end{bmatrix} \quad (3.26)$$

Considering scatter contribution incoming from more than one depth layer:

$$\mathbf{d}_{s_j} = [\mathbf{S}_j\ \mathbf{S}_{j\text{-}1} \ldots \mathbf{S}_1\ ]\ [\mathbf{I}_1\ \ \mathbf{I}_2 \ldots \mathbf{I}_j\ ]^{\mathrm{T}}\ \mathbf{b} \quad (3.27)$$

where $\mathbf{d}_{s_j}$ is the total scattered dose at depth layer j, $\mathbf{S}_i$, i=1, ... j are symmetric matrices with the corresponding elements satisfying $s_{ij}(j) > s_{ij}(j\text{-}1)$, where $s_{ij}(j)$ denotes the ij^{th} element of $\mathbf{S}_j$, with $\mathbf{S}_1$=**0**. $\mathbf{I}_i$, i=1, ...j are $n\times n$ identity matrices and **b** is the IMB vector in which the elements b_i, i=1, ...n represent the elemental intensities associated with each pencil beam.

Repeating the procedure for each pencil beam and for each preceding layer emitting and receiving scatter, it can be shown that the overall scattered contribution is given as follows:

$$\begin{bmatrix} \mathbf{d}_{s_1} \\ \mathbf{d}_{s_2} \\ \mathbf{d}_{s_3} \\ \vdots \\ \mathbf{d}_{s_m} \end{bmatrix} = \begin{bmatrix} \mathbf{S}_1 & \mathbf{0} & \mathbf{0} & \cdots & \mathbf{0} \\ \mathbf{S}_2 & \mathbf{S}_1 & \mathbf{0} & \cdots & \mathbf{0} \\ \mathbf{S}_3 & \mathbf{S}_2 & \mathbf{S}_1 & \mathbf{0} & \mathbf{0} \\ \vdots & \ddots & \ddots & \ddots & \vdots \\ \mathbf{S}_m & \cdots & \mathbf{S}_3 & \mathbf{S}_2 & \mathbf{S}_1 \end{bmatrix} \begin{bmatrix} \mathbf{I}_1 \\ \mathbf{I}_2 \\ \mathbf{I}_3 \\ \vdots \\ \mathbf{I}_m \end{bmatrix} \mathbf{b} \qquad \mathbf{d}_s = \mathbf{S}\,\tilde{\mathbf{I}}\,\mathbf{b} \quad (3.28)$$

where the $\mathbf{d}_{s_j}$, j=1...m, are the scatter dose vectors of dimension $n\times 1$ representing the scatter contribution from the cells of the jth layer at depth $x = j\Delta x$, and the sub-matrices $\mathbf{S}_j$ of dimension $n\times n$ describe the scattered contributions from the jth layer.

Remark: For a parallel beam matrix symmetrical with respect to the central axis, only n components are required to construct a $n\times n$ elemental scatter matrix $\mathbf{S}_j$, j=1...m. It follows that the elemental scatter matrices are toeplitz matrices [117] and this may be exploited to advantage in terms of efficient computation.

Making use of the superposition principle, the total dose is given by the sum of primary dose $\mathbf{d}_p$ from (3.9) and scattered dose $\mathbf{d}_s$ from (3.28) such that

$$\mathbf{d} = \mathbf{Pb} + \mathbf{S}\,\tilde{\mathbf{I}}\,\mathbf{b} \tag{3.29}$$

In practice it follows that a tuning parameter is required in order to account for variation in field size. Unlike the initial formulation, which required the use of a several tuning parameters at different depths, the modified formulation requires a single scalar tuning parameter, denoted γ. It is implemented such that

$$\mathbf{d} = \mathbf{Pb} + \gamma\mathbf{S}\,\tilde{\mathbf{I}}\,\mathbf{b} \tag{3.30}$$

or

$$\mathbf{d} = \mathbf{Pb} + \gamma\mathbf{S}\,\tilde{\mathbf{I}}\,\mathbf{b} \tag{3.31}$$

Defining the total dose calculation matrix

$$\mathbf{\Phi} = (\mathbf{P} + \gamma\mathbf{S}\,\tilde{\mathbf{I}}\,) \tag{3.32}$$

in a similar manner to the initial formulation, the dose due to a set of intensity modulated beams **b** may be expressed as:

$$\mathbf{d} = \mathbf{\Phi}\,\mathbf{b} \tag{3.33}$$

in which the tuning parameter γ is typically less than unity. For example, in order to match the measured CAX data from Walsgrave, $\gamma = 0.3$ for a 6 MV beam and $\gamma = 0.5$ for a 25 MV beam both of which having a field size of 10×10 cm.

The advantage of the modified approach is that only one scaling factor γ is required to tune the beam model as opposed to the initial model which required a scaling vector, with one element being associated with each depth.

3.3 Divergent Pencil Beam Matrix Formulation

In practice all beams exhibit divergent ray line characteristics. For head and neck cancer, where the body volume to be irradiated is small, divergence effects are found to be negligible and assumptions on parallel pencil beams lead to satisfactory results [3, 7, 8, 37, 101, 102]. When dealing with the pelvic region, however, where the beam may traverse 15 - 45 cm of the body structures, it is necessary to take into account the effect of divergence. In order to accommodate this a divergent matrix beam model, which is closer to the actual beam characteristics, is required to be developed.

It is shown that there are basically two ways in which to accommodate and make use of divergent beams. The first is to work back from a parallel pencil matrix model to find a divergent beam having a smaller field size but the same coverage or overlay of the PTA; see mapping transformation in [1]. The second approach is to pre-warp the ROIs, so that parallel beams may be utilised and, by making use of the mapping transformation, proceed by effectively mapping a divergent beam onto a parallel grid (see Sect. 3.3.1).

3.3.1 Divergent Pencil Beam Matrix Grid

It has been seen in Sect. 2.3 that actual X-ray photon beams are divergent and not parallel. However, the advantage of the pencil beam model formulation is that it is applicable to both ideal parallel beams, assuming an ideal source, and divergent or fan beams. The only difference is in the representation of the beam path. When use is made of divergent IMBs, a fan or divergent beam dose matrix representation is used (see Fig. 3.5).

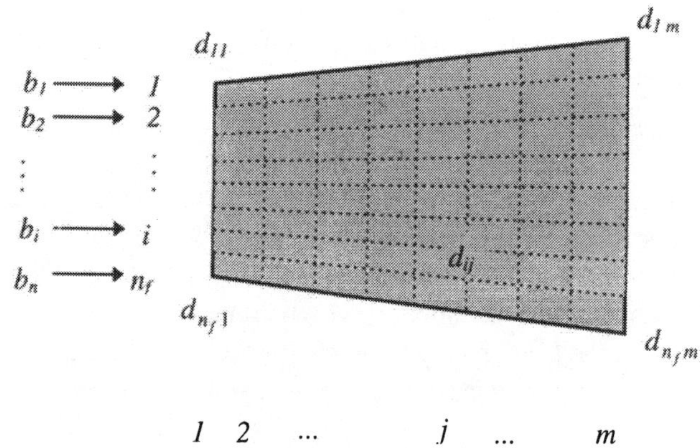

Fig. 3.5 Divergent beam dose calculation matrix

Similar to the parallel representation, each grid point lies at the intersection of a pencil beam with vertical depth lines. In Fig. 3.5 it can be observed that the pencil ray lines on the edge of the field travel a larger distance into the body than the pencil ray line lying on the central axis. This is required to be taken into account in the calculation of the primary component of the dose (see Sect. 3.3.2). Similarly, the spacings between neighbouring elemental points of the matrix increase with depth. This is also required to be taken into account in the calculation of the scatter component (see Sect. 3.3.2).

It can also be observed that the field size of the divergent beam is smaller on the patient surface than it is deeper into the body. Therefore in order to cover all the PTA a smaller field size is required when the beam is assumed to be divergent. Assuming that the spacing of the IMBs (i.e. Δy) remains the same as for a parallel beam at the point of beam entry, or patient surface, the number of IMBs for a divergent beam n_f is reduced: $n_f \leq n$. Later it is shown that this observation prompts the need to map the beam profile resulting from the optimisation of the parallel beam onto the profile used within the algorithm to optimise the divergent beam (see hybrid approach of Chap. 6). Alternatively, it is possible to keep the number of IMBs fixed with respect to the parallel beam at the point of beam entry by reducing the spacing between each divergent pencil ray line, such that $n_f = n$. Note that the number of elemental depth layers considered (i.e. the number of columns of the beam dose matrix) remains the same for both parallel and divergent beam models.

When a divergent beam is considered, use can be made of a mapping transformation detailed in [1]. This transformation 'warps' the ROIs and the PTA inside the path of the divergent beam so that the divergent pencil beams are transformed into parallel pencil beams.

Use of such a transformation enables the field size to be determined in a similar way to the method used for purely parallel beams (i.e. projecting the PTA onto the patient surface). This transformation could also be used to determine the intersection points between the OARs and parallel ray lines instead of having to calculate the trajectory of divergent ray lines with the original ROIs and OARs (see Fig. 3.6).

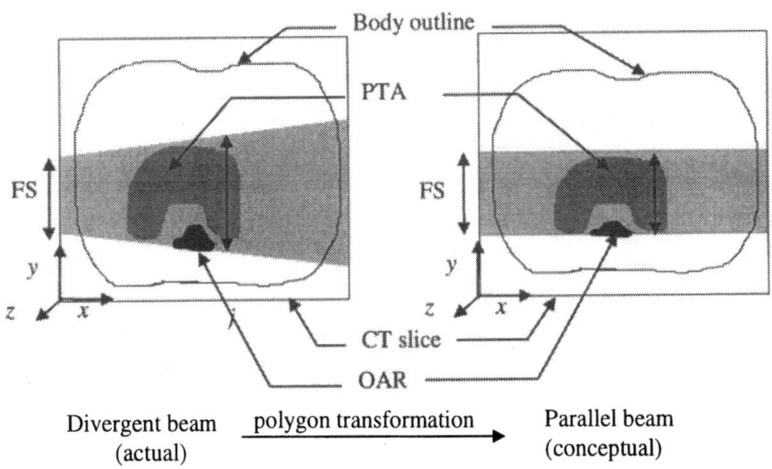

Fig. 3.6 Use of the polygon mapping transformation to determine the field size of a fan beam

A summary of the various options to deal with parallel and divergent beams is given in Table 3.1.

Table 3.1 Comparison between alternative approaches to determine intersection between ROIs and PTA with IMB ray lines

Type of beam	Description of ray lines and body polygons	
Parallel beam (Ideal)	Parallel IMB ray lines	Original ROIs and PTA
Divergent beam (Actual)	Divergent IMB ray lines	Original ROIs and PTA
Pseudo parallel beam (Conceptual)	Parallel IMB ray lines	Warped ROIs and PTA

3.3.2 Overall Divergent Dose Calculation Matrix

For a divergent beam, the form of the overall dose has the same structure as for a parallel pencil beam,
i.e.

$$\overline{\mathbf{d}} = (\overline{\mathbf{P}} + \gamma\overline{\mathbf{S}}\tilde{\mathbf{I}})\mathbf{b} \tag{3.34}$$

where the partitioned matrices $\overline{\mathbf{P}}$ and $\overline{\mathbf{S}}$ are modified to take into account the increased length of the ray lines off the central axis, thus increasing attenuation. In terms of scatter, the scattering angle also increases with depth, thereby reducing the effect of scatter with depth.

The equations relating the primary dose and the scattered dose are modified as follows:

Primary dose

$$\overline{p}(x) = x_{\max} e^{(-c_3(\overline{x}-x_{\max}))} - c_4\overline{x} + c_5\overline{x}^2 + c_6 \tag{3.35}$$

with $\overline{x}$ being the modified depth to account for the pencil beam divergence, such that:

$$\overline{x} = \frac{x}{\cos\left(\sin^{-1}\left(\frac{y}{SSD}\right)\right)} \tag{3.36}$$

where x is the equivalent depth for a parallel pencil beam, y is the distance from the central axis and SSD is the source to skin distance.

Scatter dose

The scatter component of the dose is calculated by making use of equation (3.24)

$$s_i = \frac{e^{-\sigma(r\sin(\theta))^2}}{r} \tag{3.37}$$

where

$$r = ((x_3 - x_1)^2 + (y_3 - y_1)^2)^{0.5} \tag{3.38}$$

and, by making use of the cosine rule, see Fig. 3.7,

$$\theta = \cos^{-1}\left(\frac{b^2 + c^2 - a^2}{2bc}\right) \tag{3.39}$$

with $b = r$, $a = \sqrt{(x_3 - x_2)^2 + (y_3 - y_2)^2}$ and $c = \sqrt{(x_2 - x_1)^2 + (y_2 - y_1)^2}$

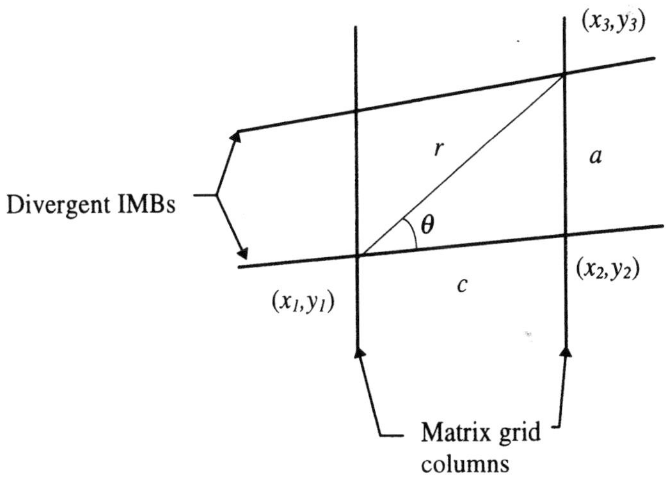

Fig. 3.7 Illustrating geometry of divergent beam scatter

From these relationships the matrices $\overline{\mathbf{P}}$ and $\overline{\mathbf{S}}$ may be deduced, i.e. $\overline{\mathbf{P}} = f_p(\theta)$ and $\overline{\mathbf{S}} = f_s(\theta)$, where f_p and f_s are functions of the divergent geometry of the pencil beams. Note that each scatter sub-matrix $\overline{\mathbf{S}}_j$, $j=1...m$, is required to be calculated independently. This leads to an increase in complexity in terms of additional computation.

3.4 Inclusion of In-Air-Profile, Penumbra and Patient Contour Correction

In-air-profile (IAP), penumbra and patient contour all affect the beam profiles. These effects have been accommodated into the beam models, with use being made of matrix multiplication between 'masking' matrices and the vector of IMBs. The masking matrices are diagonal and the diagonal elements relate to the profiles for the IAP, the penumbra and patient specific correction factors to account for non flat patient contours. The following subsections show how these practical factors are included into the developed beam models.

3.4.1 Inclusion of the IAP

The IAP affects all the IMBs associated with a particular beam. Therefore it is necessary to pre-multiply each set of IMBs by its respective IAP scaling factor. This can be implemented via a product between a diagonal matrix $\mathbf{M}_{iap}$, containing the IAP scaling factors on the diagonal, and the IMB vector $\mathbf{b}$ such that the modified beam profile denoted $\mathbf{b}'$ is given by:

$$\begin{bmatrix} b'_1 \\ b'_2 \\ \vdots \\ b'_n \end{bmatrix} = \begin{bmatrix} v_{iap\,1} & 0 & \cdots & 0 \\ 0 & v_{iap\,2} & \ddots & \vdots \\ \vdots & \ddots & \ddots & 0 \\ 0 & \cdots & 0 & v_{iap\,n} \end{bmatrix} \begin{bmatrix} b_1 \\ b_2 \\ \vdots \\ b_n \end{bmatrix} \tag{3.40}$$

i.e.

$$\mathbf{b}' = \mathbf{M}_{iap}\,\mathbf{b} \tag{3.41}$$

3.4.2 Inclusion of Patient Contour Correction

Assuming no in-air scatter interaction between the pencil beams, the in-air attenuation of an X-ray beam is inversely proportional to the square of the distance [53]. When the beam encounters non flat patient contours it is necessary to make use of patient contour correction procedures within the beam calculation algorithm. The dose on the patient surface is a maximum when the source to skin distance (SSD) is a minimum, i.e. $\mathrm{SSD}_{\min}$. The attenuation of the elemental pencil beam at this point is normalised to unity, so that the normalised attenuation coefficients, denoted $v_{cont}(i)$, i=1..n, for the other pencil beams are given by $v_{cont}(i) = \mathrm{SSD}_{\min}^2 / \mathrm{SSD}_i^2$, i.e. the ratio of the square of the distances travelled from the source to the patient SSD_i with respect to $\mathrm{SSD}_{\min}$.

Similarly this can be implemented via a product between a diagonal matrix $\mathbf{M}_{cont}$, containing the attenuation factors for the patient contour correction on the diagonal, and the modified IMB vector **b'** such that a new modified beam profile **b"** is given by:

$$\begin{bmatrix} b''_1 \\ b''_2 \\ \vdots \\ b''_n \end{bmatrix} = \begin{bmatrix} v_{cont\,1} & 0 & \cdots & 0 \\ 0 & v_{cont\,2} & \ddots & \vdots \\ \vdots & \ddots & \ddots & 0 \\ 0 & \cdots & 0 & v_{cont\,n} \end{bmatrix} \begin{bmatrix} b'_1 \\ b'_2 \\ \vdots \\ b'_n \end{bmatrix} \tag{3.42}$$

i.e.

$$\mathbf{b}'' = \mathbf{M}_{cont}\,\mathbf{b}' \tag{3.43}$$

3.4.3 Inclusion of the Penumbra

Accounting for the penumbra involves modifying the dose on the edge of the field. This is achieved by assuming a beam matrix larger than necessary so that it includes the penumbra region. In this region, the IMBs are modified by an attenuation factor obtained from the use of the polynomial function given in Chap. 2, Sect. 2.4.3. In order to accommodate for the overall dimension of the IMB vector, IMBs that are not affected by the penumbra are not modified. This is achieved by multiplying unaffected pencil beams by a unity factor. Again this is implemented by multiplying the previously modified IMB vector **b"** by a diagonal matrix $\mathbf{M}_{pen}$ in which diagonal elements are either equal to unity or to the attenuation factor such that:

$$\begin{bmatrix} b'''_1 \\ \vdots \\ b'''_{h-1} \\ b'''_h \\ \vdots \\ b'''_{i-1} \\ b'''_i \\ \vdots \\ b'''_n \end{bmatrix} = \begin{bmatrix} v_{pen_1} & & & & & & & \\ & \ddots & & & & \mathbf{0} & & \\ & & v_{pen_h} & & & & & \\ & & & 1 & & & & \\ & & & & \ddots & & & \\ & & & & & 1 & & \\ & & \mathbf{0} & & & & v_{pen_i} & & \\ & & & & & & & \ddots & \\ & & & & & & & & v_{pen_n} \end{bmatrix} \begin{bmatrix} b''_1 \\ \vdots \\ b''_{h-1} \\ b''_h \\ \vdots \\ b''_{i-1} \\ b''_i \\ \vdots \\ b''_n \end{bmatrix} \tag{3.44}$$

i.e.

$$\mathbf{b}''' = \mathbf{M}_{pen}\,\mathbf{b}'' \tag{3.45}$$

3.4.4 General Formulation of the Matrix Based Beam Model

Incorporation of the factors in Sect. 3.4.1, 3.4.2 and 3.4.3 leads to an expression for the modified total dose vector as a function of the IMB vector as follows:

Parallel beam

$$\mathbf{d} = (\mathbf{P} + \gamma \mathbf{S}\,\tilde{\mathbf{I}})(\mathbf{M}_{pen}(\mathbf{M}_{cont}(\mathbf{M}_{iap}\mathbf{b}))) \tag{3.46}$$

Divergent beam

$$\bar{\mathbf{d}} = (\bar{\mathbf{P}} + \gamma\bar{\mathbf{S}}\tilde{\mathbf{I}})\,(\mathbf{M}_{pen}(\mathbf{M}_{cont}(\mathbf{M}_{iap}\mathbf{b}))) \tag{3.47}$$

3.5 Verification and Tuning of Developed Beam Model

The assessment of any beam model involves the comparison between measured and calculated data. In order to make use of the beam model in a clinical environment, to predict and deliver conformal treatment, the beam model has been tuned to replicate measured data for the particular machines considered. In this section the measured dose data are represented by '+++' whilst the calculated dose data are represented by solid lines. At Walsgrave Hospital two linacs have been selected to deliver conformal treatment; namely a 6 MV and a 25 MV photon beam. The 6 MV linac is used primarily for treatment of tumours close to the beam entry point whilst the 25 MV linac is usually used to treat cancer located at a greater depth, such as the bladder in the pelvic region.

Note that compensators are situated on a tray at some 66 cm from the source (34 cm from the patient), therefore, in order to deliver a 10 cm by 10 cm intensity modulated beam, it is necessary to produce a 6.6 cm by 6.6 cm compensator with a profile of various height.

Experimental set up. Measurements were conducted at Walsgrave Hospital with use being made of a water phantom. A water phantom (see Fig. 3.9) is composed of a water tank of cubical shape of dimension 60×60×60 cm. Two ionisation chambers are used to measure the dose profiles in water. The first ionisation chamber, used as a reference, measures the exposure in air for the non-attenuated beam, above the compensators. The second ionisation chamber measures the exposure in water at different depths. It is fixed on guides that can be moved by four DC motors in three directions x, y and z, inside the water tank, where x is the length, y is the width and z is the height. In order to assess the 2-D beam model, measurements were performed along the x axis at different heights or depths. The procedure for tuning the beam model consists of:

- matching the CAX %DD
- measuring penumbra and deducing a fifth order polynomial

– using data from the treatment planning system to approximate the IAP
– tuning the σ_i and γ (see equation 3.21 and 3.28) to match the experimental data

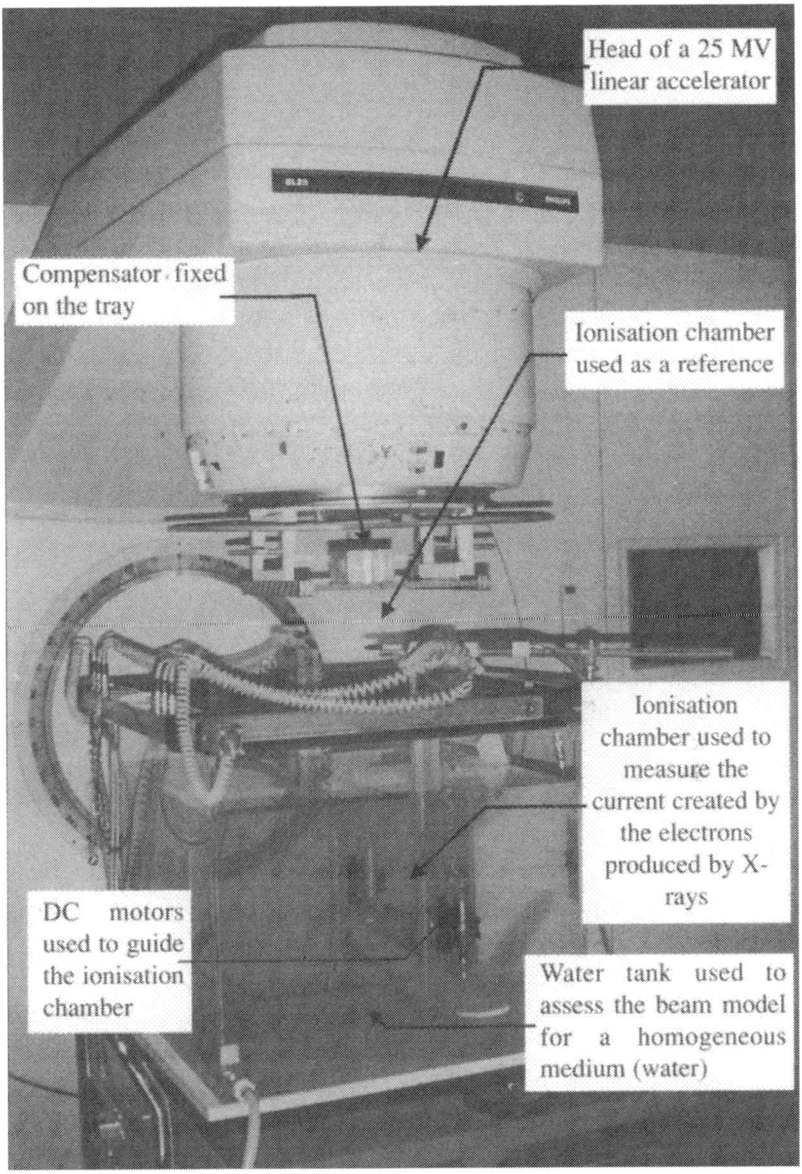

Fig. 3.8 Water tank used to assess the beam model for a homogeneous medium, courtesy of Walsgrave Hospital, NHS Trust, Coventry

3.5.1 Open Field Tests

Central Axis. The behaviour of a beam interacting with the human body structure can be described or characterised by its CAX %DD and its profile at various depths. This gives information regarding the attenuation of the beam with respect to depth, whilst the beam profile characterises the variation of the dose across the field.

A simplified version of the developed beam model has previously been favourably compared to standard %DD given in the Supplement 17 of the British Journal of Radiology [25] for 6 MV photon beams [106, 108]. The model developed in this work consistently shows good agreement between calculated dose and standard dose representing the average output of a 6 MV linear accelerator for photon beams [108]. Note that these tests necessarily involve the divergent beam model. This provided the confidence to subsequently tune the beam model to the particular accelerators used at Walsgrave Hospital.

For each machine the CAX %DD has been measured with an ionisation chamber immersed in a water phantom. The process involved measuring the dosage whereby the ionisation chamber is moved along the beam central axis between depths x=0 and x=30 cm. The accuracy of the measurements depends on several factors such as the location of the ionisation chamber with respect to the actual beam central axis, the size of the ionisation chamber (here 4 mm) and its ability to measure accurately the ionisation that takes place. All these errors, which can be due to the dosimeter physical characteristics and/or to human factors, are combined together to form an experimental error which is assumed to be within ±5% for all the measurements involving the water phantom. It has been shown in Chap. 2, Fig. 2.3, that the calculated CAX %DD from the model leads to a good agreement with the measured data for both the 6 MV and 25 MV photon beams, with the difference between the measured and the calculated dose being within ±1%. Such an error level is considered as acceptable as it is well within experimental error. The CAX % DD of Fig. 2.3 is reproduced for completeness here as Fig. 3.9.

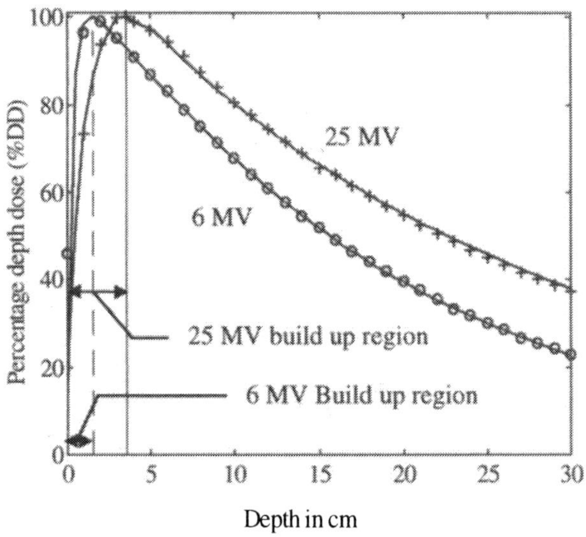

Fig. 3.9 Central axis percentage depth dose for 6 MV ('o' measured, '-' calculated) and 25 MV photon beams ('+' measured, '-' calculated)

Scatter Component. In the approach developed, primary and scatter components of the dose are separated. Figures 3.10 and 3.11 represent 3-D plots of the scatter component for a 6 MV and a 25 MV parallel pencil beams respectively. For both beam energies, the scatter is shown to increase with depth, with its maximum contribution lying on the central axis.

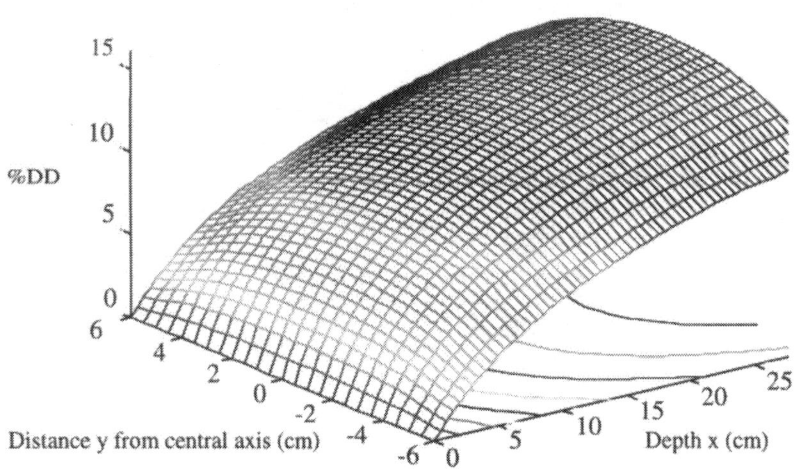

Fig. 3.10 Scatter component for a 6 MV photon beam with a 10×10 cm FS

It can be observed that for the 25 MV beam (see Fig. 3.11), that the amount of scatter in the build up region is initially zero. This is due to the assumption in the model that the dose in the build up region is only due to primary up to (x_{max}-1.5) cm*. Note that whilst this assumption is not based on physical considerations, as the build up region in fact arises due to the flow of charged particles created by the interaction of photons with mater [53] (see Sect. 3.4.1), it does however, allow the overall beam characteristic to be replicated.

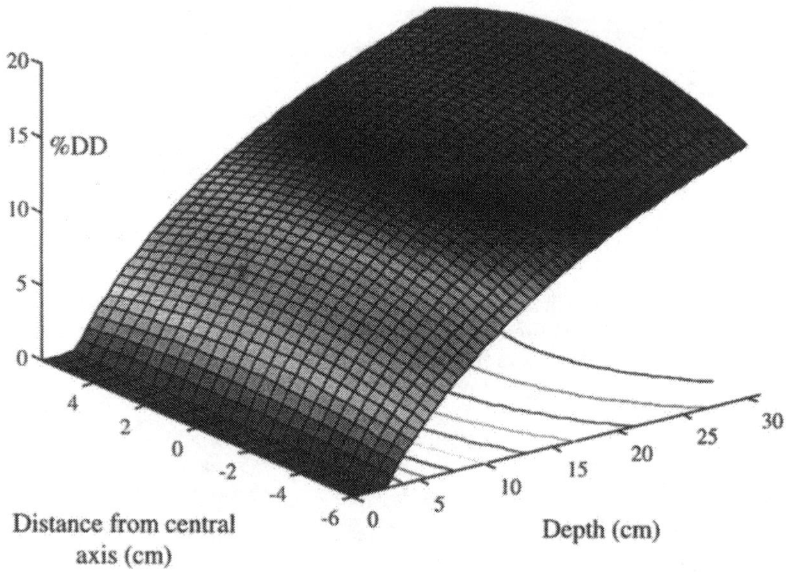

Fig. 3.11: Scatter component for a 25 MV photon beam with a 10×10 cm FS

Primary Contribution and Total Contribution. The scatter component is then added to the primary component to give the total dose, see Fig. 3.12, which shows isodose plots characteristics for 6 MV and 25 MV beams assuming parallel pencil beams. Note that at the point of equilibrium, the IAP produces a concave profile. As the depth increases, the beam profile becomes more convex, see the total isodose plots of Figures 3.12(b) and 3.12(d), whereas the isodose plots for the primary contribution remain concave, see Fig. 3.12(a) and 3.12(c).

Isodose plots are given for %DD = {100, 95, 90, 70, 60, 50, 40, 30, 20, 10} with the maximum dose normalised at the point of equilibrium. Note that the 25 MV photon beam is less attenuated than the 6 MV photon beam.

---

* Recall that the location of x_{max} is approximately 1.5 cm for a 6 MV and 3.5 cm for a 25 MV, see Sect. 2.4.1.

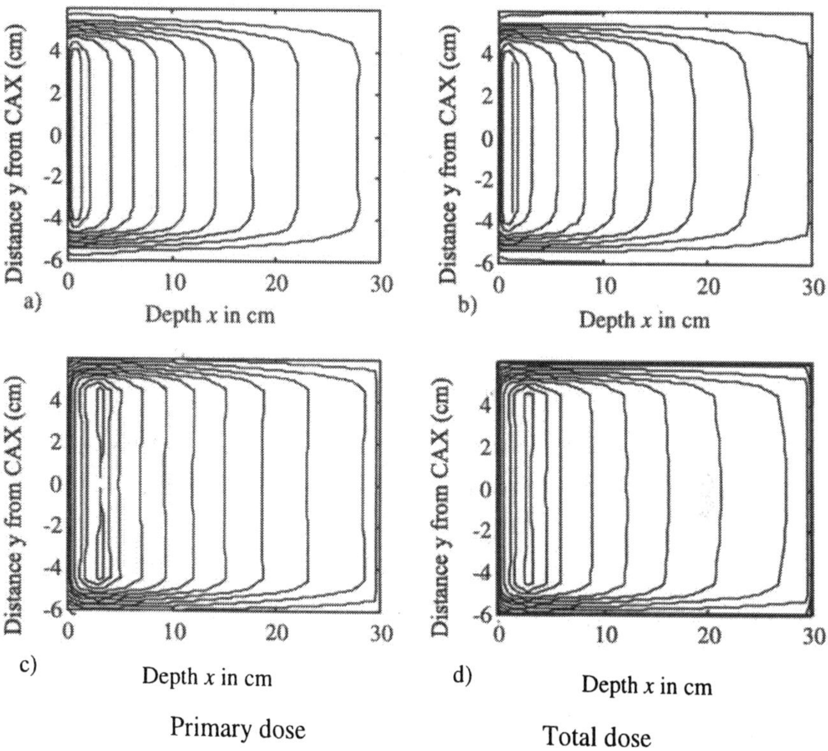

Fig. 3.12 Comparison between primary and total dose for parallel beams tuned to replicate measured data for a 6 MV beam (upper) and a 25 MV beam (lower)

Influence of Inhomogeneities on a 6 MV Beam With a 10 cm × 10 cm Field Size. Although the ability of the model to replicate inhomogeneities has not been assessed against measured data due to the unavailability of an inhomogeneous phantom, the results from the simulation of inhomogeneous media is shown in Fig. 3.13, and 3.14 for completeness. Figure 3.13 shows the %DD along a pencil beam path located at -2 cm from the central axis and Fig. 3.14 shows the corresponding isodose plot.

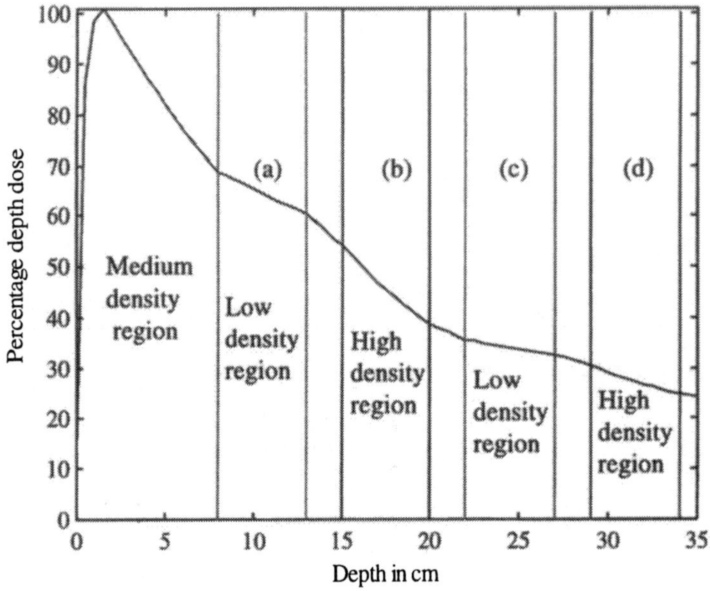

Fig. 3.13 Percentage depth dose along a pencil beam path located at -2 cm from the central axis

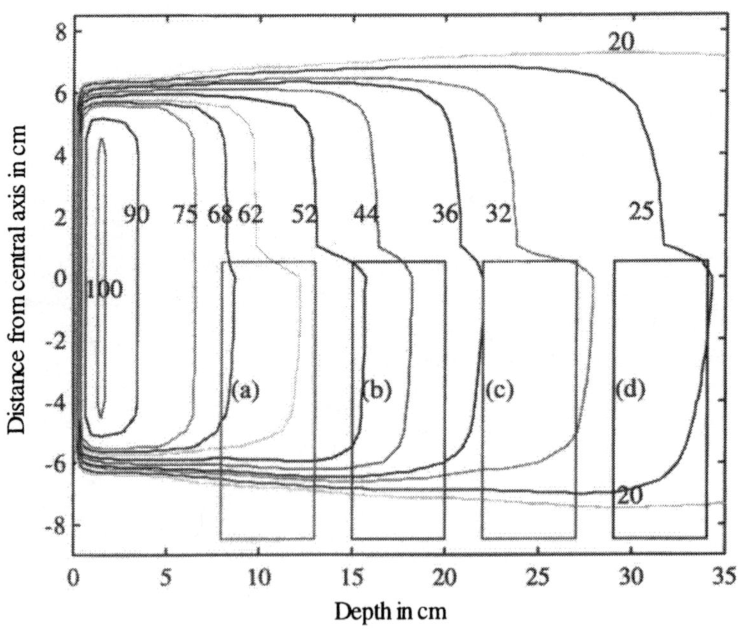

Fig. 3.14 Isodose contour plot to visualise the influence of inhomogeneities

The inhomogeneity regions are represented by rectangular shaped areas (a), (b), (c) and (d), of which (a) and (c) represent regions of lower densities than the normal body density (similar to water), with (b) and (d) being regions of higher densities (see Chap. 2, section 2.4). Recalling section 2.4.5, the linear attenuation coefficient for the normal body structure, the low density region and the high density region are given by μ_1 = 0.06 cm^{-1}, μ_2 = 0.03 cm^{-1} and μ_3 = 0.09 cm^{-1} respectively. As opposed to the previous set of results, the beam calculation and display algorithms make use of the divergent beam model.

Note that although the effect of inhomogeneities is shown only for a 6 MV beam, it can also be taken into account in the case of 25 MV beam when inhomogeneous media are considered.

Beam Profile Information on the beam profiles have been obtained by measuring the beam profiles for a 6 MV beam with a 10 cm by 10 cm open field (with no blocking material inserted in the beam path) at depths x of 1.5, 5.0, 9.5, 14.0, 20.0, 25.0, and 29.0 cm. The resulting characteristics, shown in Fig. 3.15, represent the isodose distributions obtained from the measured and calculated dose data. Note that in all cases the doses were calculated with use being made of the divergent beam model.

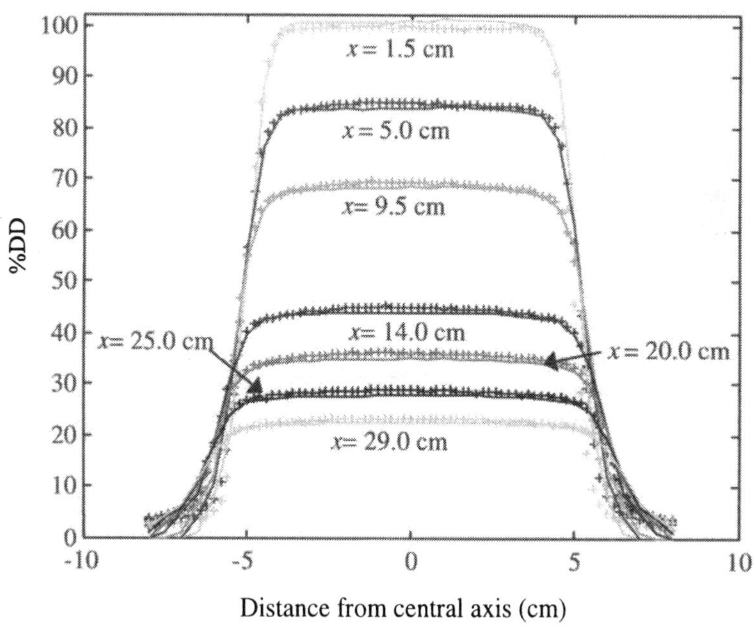

Fig. 3.15 Comparison between measured '+' and calculated '-' dose distribution represented by isodose plots at 1.5, 5.0, 9.5, 14.0, 20.0, 25.0, and 29.0 cm depth for a 6 MV 10 cm by 10 cm open field

For the central part of the beam, the model is able to adequately replicate the measured dose and, as has been shown in Chap. 2, is found to have a mean error of approximately 1.6%. The dose modelled in the lower part of the penumbra region is however not as accurate, with an error in terms of percentage depth dose of approximately 3%, some of this error being due to the mapping process which transforms a parallel beam into a divergent beam. Note that additional errors are also introduced when rotating the beam dose matrix mapping it onto the reference grid. However, these errors could be reduced by making use of a finer resolution. Overall, the level of accuracy is considered to be sufficient to demonstrate the efficacy of the developed optimisation routines, see Chap. 4 and 5.

3.5.2 Intensity Modulated Beams

Guaranteeing a good agreement between measured and calculated dose data for an open field is not sufficient for ensuring that the beam model is able to replicate an intensity modulated beam dose distribution. In order to demonstrate the ability of the model to replicate the behaviour of intensity modulated beams, lead compensators of various shapes have been inserted into an actual beam path. Profile measurements have then been recorded at several different depths, including x_{max} = 1.5 cm, which provides the original beam profile. This is used as the input of the beam model and, as a consequence, is used as a reference for the measurements of the various compensators.

Thin Lead Compensator. A lead compensator shown in Fig. 3.16, positioned on a tray produces the dose distribution profiles shown in Fig. 3.17. This compensator could be used to correct for some small inhomogeneity and/or non flat patient contours.

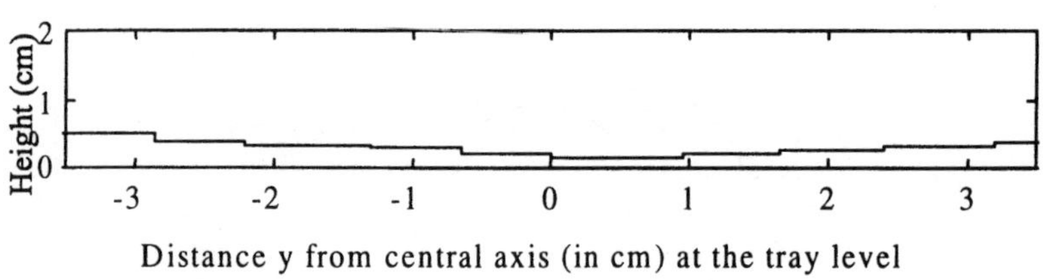

Fig. 3.16 Compensator profile

The resulting beam profiles at 1.5, 9.5, 14.0, 25.0 and 29.0 cm depth show good agreement between measured and calculated dose data. The mean absolute error expressed as a percentage between the calculated and the measured dose is approximately 1.9% which is slightly higher than for an open field (1.6%). The dose discrepancy on the very edge of the field is found to be larger i.e. ±2% in terms of percentage depth dose. However, the level of dose discrepancy is considered to be of minor importance as it concerns regions on the very edge of the field which account for less than 5% of the maximum dose delivered by the particular beam considered.

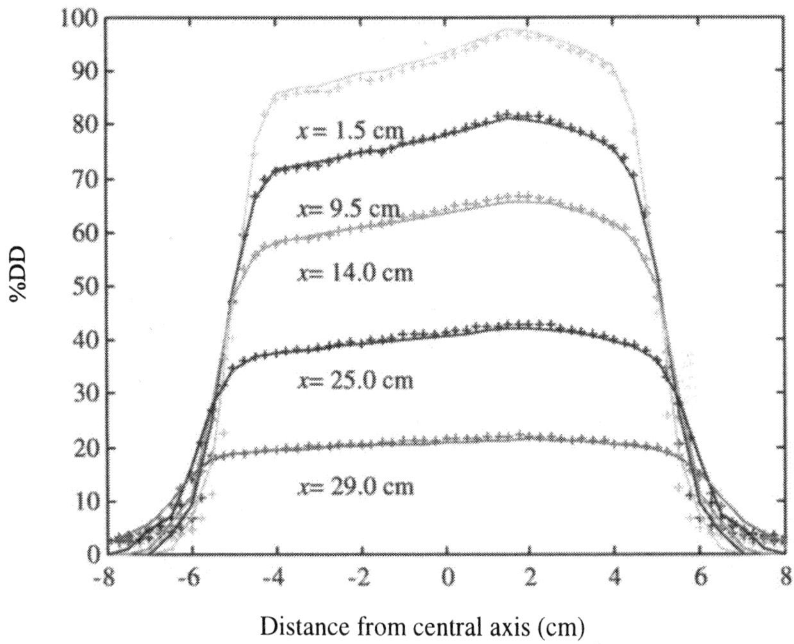

Fig. 3.17 Comparison between measured '+' and calculated '-' dose distribution represented by isodose plots at 1.5, 9.5, 14.0, 25.0 and 29.0 cm depth for a 6 MV photon beam (10 cm by 10 cm field size) with a thin lead compensator inserted into the beam path

Note that although the lead compensator is manufactured such that it comprises small 'discrete' steps in its profile, the isodose plot shown in Fig. 3.17 indicates continuous graduation. This is due to the scatter interaction (i.e. filtering action) that takes place within the compensators. This practical aspect is of particular importance in the realisation of IMBs determined by simulation (see Chap. 4, and 6).

Wedge Shaped Compensators. Figure 3.18 shows a wedge shaped compensator that is shorter than the field size for which it is inserted. The dose is observed to decrease gradually on the left side of the field then increases relatively sharply, due to the absence of any compensating material on the edges of the field (see Fig. 3.19). Again the model is able to reproduce the dose distribution adequately with the mean absolute error expressed as a percentage between the calculated and the measured dose being 1.8%. This is comparable to the results obtained using the thin lead compensator. The dose discrepancy on the very edge of the field is within ±3% in terms of percentage depth dose.

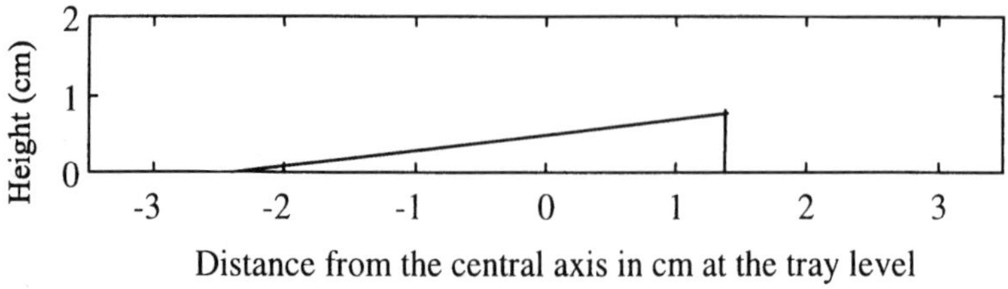

Fig. 3.18 Wedge shaped compensator profile for a wedge smaller than the field size

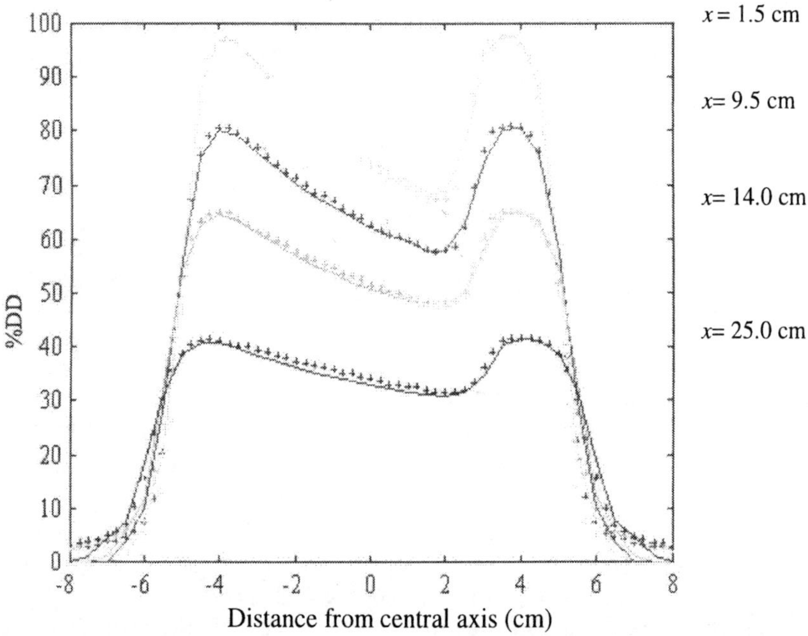

Fig. 3.19 Comparison between measured '+' and calculated '-' dose distribution represented by isodose plots at 1.5, 9.5, 14.0 and 25.0 depth for a 6 MV photon beam (10 cm by 10 cm field size) with a wedge shaped compensator inserted into the beam path

Note that although the wedge shaped compensator has a vertical edge between the highest point of the compensator and the tray, the isodose plots show a much smoother increase of the dose. This limits the type of profile that can be physically achieved with patient specific compensators. This is required to be taken into account in the optimisation process as well as in the implementation (see Chap. 4 and 6).

Triangular shaped compensator. Figure 3.20 shows a triangular shaped compensator inserted into the beam path and positioned on a tray such that the highest point of the compensator lies on the beam central axis. The resulting dose distribution represented by beam profiles measured at 1.5, 9.5, 14.0, 25.0 and 29.0 cm depth show good agreement between measured and calculated dose data (see Fig. 3.21).

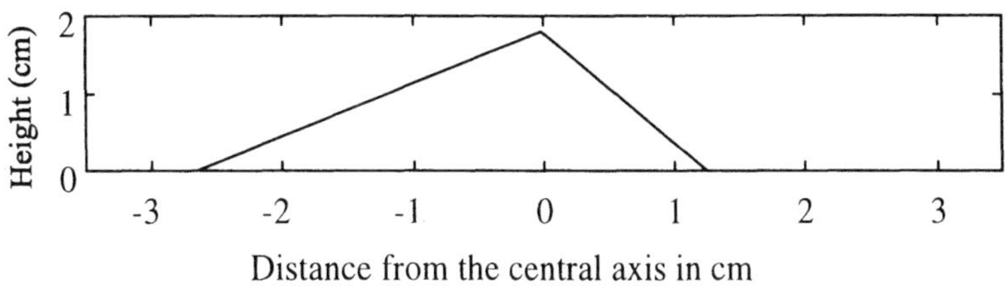

Fig. 3.20 Triangular compensator profile

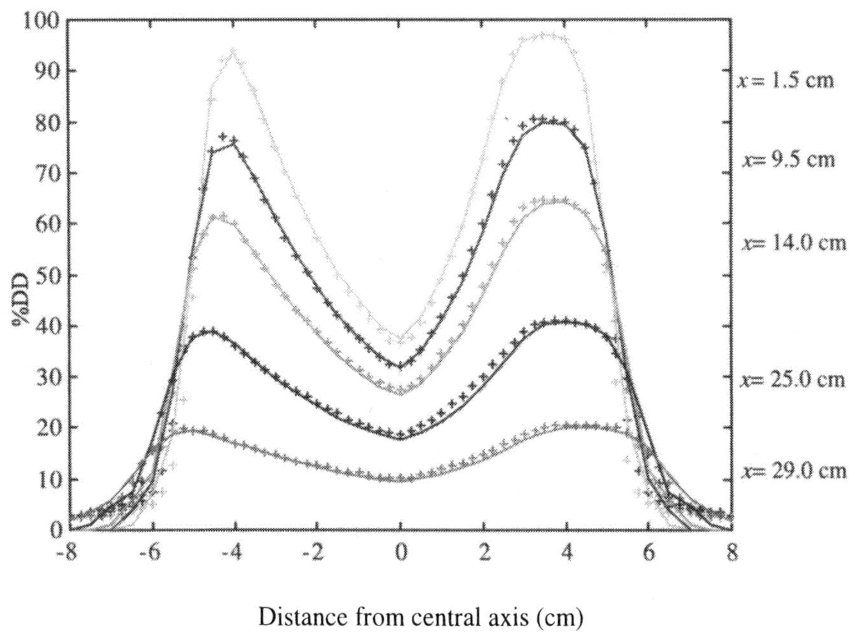

Fig. 3.21 Comparison between measured (+) and calculated (-) dose distribution represented by isodose plots at 1.5, 9.5, 14.0, 25.0 and 29.0 cm depth for a 6 MV photon beam (10 cm by 10 cm field size) with a triangular shaped compensator inserted into the beam path

As expected, the highest attenuation occurs on the beam CAX, with the gradient of the triangular shaped compensator determining the slope of the beam profiles from the CAX to the edges of the field. Again a satisfactory agreement between measured and calculated dose is achieved (mean absolute error of 2.5% in the central part of the beam and about ±3% in terms of percentage depth dose on the bottom edge of the field). It is interesting to note that the dose discrepancy increases as the gradient of the compensator increases. This is due to the fact that the scatter contribution from the high dose region within the beam is slightly underestimated.

3.6 Concluding remarks

Building on the physical characteristics and preliminary modelling considerations introduced in Chap. 2, Chap. 3 has developed a matrix based beam model which enables the individual modelling of elementary pencil beams. This is a fundamental step in the development of optimisation algorithms for conformational therapy since the notion of pencil beams is synonymous with that of intensity modulated beams (IMBs); thus the modelling of IMBs is now possible.

The approach has followed the development of a parallel pencil beam since this is a simpler concept and is a special case of the more general divergent beam. Having established the basis of the parallel beam, the extension to the divergent, or fan, beam has been shown to be straightforward. It is shown later in Chap. 5 and 6 that the parallel and divergent beams lend themselves to the use of iterative least squares and genetic algorithms in the solution of the inverse problem and as a forward solving mechanism, respectively.

When taking into account the physical features introduced in Chap. 2, such as in-air-profile, penumbra, and patient contour correction, it is shown later that the resulting model produces satisfactory results [118]; although the penumbra proved to be a little difficult to replicate. However, the results were considered to be sufficiently accurate, providing confidence to continue with the developed model. The next step is to make use of the developed model in order to determine the optimum set of IMBs; this constituting the solution of the inverse problem which is considered in Chap. 4.

CHAPTER 4

SOLVING THE INVERSE PROBLEM IN RADIOTHERAPY TREATMENT PLANNING

4.1 Introduction

A complex problem such as the optimisation of radiotherapy treatment requires the simultaneous solution of multiple objectives. Excluding the ideal case, where all the objectives can be solved uniquely, the objectives are in general conflicting in nature [3, 35, 80, 101, 119]. For example in radiotherapy one objective is to deliver a high dose to the PTA, and another one is to minimise the dose delivered to the OHT. Ideally 100% dose in the PTA is required to be achieved and 0% elsewhere, but due to the physical methods employed in the delivery of radiotherapy, it is not possible to simultaneously fulfil these two objectives. This is because in order to reach the diseased regions radiation is required to pass through healthy tissues.

In addition, it is not possible to remove a radiation dose, which implies that the IMBs are required to be positive or null. Further, the production of IMBs is subject to physical and mechanical constraints due to the beam delivery mechanisms. For example, in this work, where use is made of patient specific compensators, it has been found that it is not possible to produce neighbouring IMBs with large differences in intensity. Therefore constraints on gradient between neighbouring IMBs are required to be implemented in order to produce physically realisable and medically acceptable solutions to the inverse problem.

4.2 Definition of the Inverse Problem

Recall from Chap. 1 that the so called inverse problem [3, 4, 5, 93] is concerned with the determination of a set of optimal IMBs from a dose prescription issued by a clinician. Whereas traditional techniques used by treatment planners make use of a forward solving process based on experience and good practice to modify the beam profiles (see Chap. 1), the inverse problem involves solving for the IMBs by working back from a dose prescription to determine the beam profiles that can produce such a dose distribution (see Fig. 4.1).

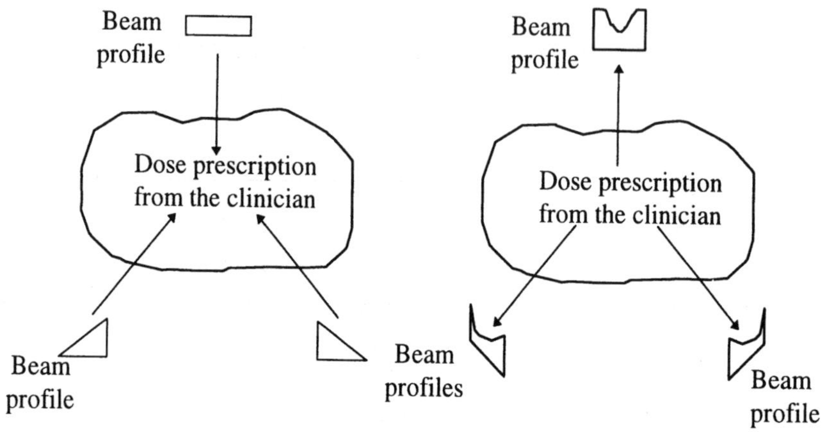

Fig. 4.1 Comparison of the forward and inverse approaches to solving the RTP problem

By adopting a control engineering perspective, the solution of the inverse problem involves modelling of the IMBs as inputs to a system, with the total dose produced by these IMBs being the output of the system. Such a model has been introduced in Chap. 2 and subsequently developed in Chap. 3. This matrix based beam model provides the means to determine the dose resulting from a particular set of inputs, i.e. the IMBs and vice versa to obtain the set of IMBs that produce a particular beam dose distribution. Such a procedure, which is analogous to the concept of designing a controller for an industrial process, forms the basis of the approach developed in this Thesis to solve the inverse problem.

4.2.1 Brief Review of Previous Approaches

The inverse problem has been solved with various methods of approach, see Chap. 1. Some are calculus or analytical based, whilst others are based on guided random search techniques such as simulated annealing, or genetic algorithms (see Chap. 5). In [120], Vance has used a GA to accommodate non linear objectives to a solution obtained when use was made of a quadratic objective function optimised using maximum entropy [100, 103]. However, whenever the optimisation method relies solely on a random based search, it has been reported that such methods may be outperformed in efficiency by other methods, referred to by Brahme in [3] as belonging to the 'systematic iterative group'. A common feature to all the previous approaches used to solve the inverse problem is the need to formulate a relationship between the IMBs and all the points in the reference grid where the dose is required to be optimised.

In previous work, see for example [3, 4, 5, 8, 102], each dose point is associated to one IMB in a one to one relationship, where there are as many inputs as there are outputs. The inputs are the set of elemental beam intensities to be determined and the outputs are the dose points to be optimised according to a given prescription. The relationship between the dose requirements and the optimum IMBs can be expressed as a set of linear equations. The one to one relationship enables the system to be well determined with a unique solution for the of IMBs. However, the dose prescription may not always be achievable, depending on the geometry of the patient together with the number of IMBs involved in the solution. Therefore, iterative optimisation procedures have been developed. The most popular techniques applied to solve the inverse problem are based on gradient search methods [2, 4]. These optimisation methods start by assuming that the function to be minimised can be expanded about its minimum as a truncated Taylor series. This involves the calculation of the first partial derivatives, i.e. the gradient, as well as the second partial derivatives, i.e. the so called Hessian [3, 72, 121, 122]. However, in order to calculate the Hessian matrix, it is necessary that the function to be optimised is twice continuously differentiable. Some of the iterative solutions resulting from these approaches require that the inverse of the Hessian matrix be computed [72, 102]. However in the context of RTP it has been reported, [67, 72, 99], that direct inversion of the Hessian matrix is usually difficult, or even impossible, and an approximation of the Hessian matrix has been employed. A comparison of the different approximations used has been reviewed by Holmes [72]. In summary, previous workers have approximated the Hessian matrix with a positive definite diagonal matrix. This has often been chosen as the identity matrix pre-multiplied by a scalar to control the speed of convergence of the algorithms [68, 80]. Making use of the approximated Hessian matrix, the solution is then refined iteratively.

4.2.2 Inverse Problem - Preliminaries

Whereas other workers have chosen a 'global' approach to the inverse problem, modelling the influence of all the IMBs on a particular plan, the approach adopted in this work considers each beam involved in the treatment semi-independently. Distinct to previous work which has involved a continuous rotation of the beam modulation apparatus about the patient, see for example [72, 73, 74, 102]; the approach adopted in this work is more specifically aimed at a static delivery of conformal plans. This involves the delivery of the treatment from a number of predetermined beam positions (see Chap. 1). It is, therefore, seen as appropriate to divide the overall inverse problem into N_{beam} individual inverse problems with the error between predicted dose and required dose being partitioned iteratively until a satisfactory solution has been achieved.

In order to remove the need to estimate, or to approximate, the second derivative involved in the solution of the inverse problem, an approach based on iterative least squares (ILS) has been adopted. This formulation exploits the features of the beam model that provides a relationship between the *nm* elements of each beam dose and *n* IMBs per beam. This differs to the previous approaches in that the system of linear equations is now over-determined and, therefore, the solution is no longer unique; the aim now being to minimise the sum of squares of the errors.

By considering each beam as a semi-independent system, it is necessary to design a methodology to superimpose the effect of each beam, so that the total dose can be obtained with a forward procedure; with the same procedure being applied in reverse to obtain the beam profiles from the dose prescription. The forward process involves the calculation of each independent dose distribution, the rotation of each beam dose matrix [1] and the superposition of the resulting beam dose matrix onto the reference grid. In order to solve the inverse problem, this procedure is required to be designed such that it is possible to work back from the overall dose prescription to individual dose prescriptions and then deduce the final optimal beam profiles. This approach is summarised in Fig. 4.2.

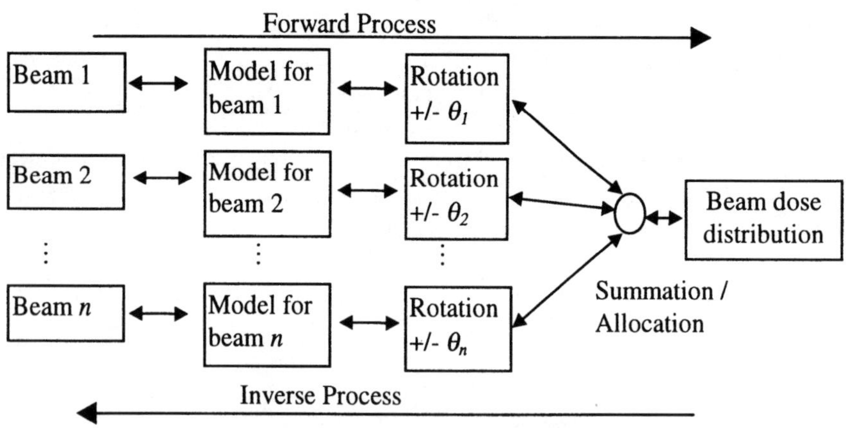

Fig. 4.2 Illustrating forward and inverse process of optimising IMBs

Such an approach has the advantage of dividing a large and computationally complex problem into N_{beam} reduced order local problems that can be solved more easily. In addition, it is possible to solve each of these problems in parallel, with the subsequent generation of the overall solution by combining the partial solutions.

When adopting this individual beam approach is it necessary to take into consideration factors influencing the allocation of a portion of the dose prescription to each beam system. In this work, although various schemes have been investigated [108] (see Sect. 4.3.2), each beam is initially allocated an equal Portion of the dose prescription, and subsequently an equal portion of the error between the dose prescription and that predicted.

4.3 Formulating the Inverse Problem for Matrix Based Beam Model

The inverse problem may be stated concisely as follows:

Given a clinical dose prescription, is it possible to work back to find an optimal set of IMBs that satisfy criteria relating to prescribed dose in the PTA whilst at the same time not exceeding dose constraints in OHT and in particular OARs?

The problem, rather like an estimation problem in control engineering, may be visualised in two stages. The first is to establish the number and orientation of the beams (analogous to selecting the structure of a transfer function) and the second stage, which builds on the first, is that of estimating/evaluating the optimum IMBs (analogous to estimating the coefficients of an assumed transfer function).

The conformational problem is essentially that of achieving a desired dosage, denoted $\tilde{\mathbf{d}}$, which relates to a treatment area defined by a treatment matrix **D** (see Chap. 3), given the relationship

$$\mathbf{d} = \boldsymbol{\Phi}\mathbf{b} \tag{4.1}$$

which relates actual (or predicted dose) resulting from the IMBs.

The problem, formulated in terms of the matrix based beam model, is to obtain a set of IMBs, i.e. **b** in order to satisfy the dose requirements $\tilde{\mathbf{d}}$ based on the beam model $\boldsymbol{\Phi} = [\mathbf{P} + \gamma\mathbf{S}\tilde{\mathbf{I}}]$ for parallel beams and $\overline{\boldsymbol{\Phi}} = \left[\overline{\mathbf{P}} + \gamma\overline{\mathbf{S}}\tilde{\mathbf{I}}\right]$ for divergent beams. In this Chap. parallel beams are considered only. The resulting dose **d** obtained from

$$\mathbf{d} = \left[\mathbf{P} + \gamma\mathbf{S}\tilde{\mathbf{I}}\right]\mathbf{b} \tag{4.2}$$

may differ from desired dose $\tilde{\mathbf{d}}$ by an amount ε, which is required to be minimised via adjustment of the IMBs in **b**.

In the context of least squares the quantity ε represents a sequence of fitting errors which includes both errors due to estimation and modelling. Since the actual error cannot be measured, only the predicted error is available for minimisation; thus reinforcing the need in the first instance for an accurate beam model for the purpose of optimisation.

4.3.1 Derivation of ILS for a Single Beam

The solution of the inverse problem is approached in this Chap. with use being made of standard least squares initially and, having established the approach as a viable method, it is then refined to the case of cautious least squares (CLS)[123] and extended to a Kalman filter type formulation [124]

In the case of a single beam, $\mathbf{b} \in \Re^n$, the basic linear least squares algorithm attempts to minimise the sum of the squares of the errors

$$\mathbf{J}_{(\mathbf{b})} = \left\{ \left[\tilde{\mathbf{d}} - \mathbf{d} \right]^{\mathrm{T}} \left[\tilde{\mathbf{d}} - \mathbf{d} \right] \right\} \tag{4.3}$$

$$\mathbf{J}_{(\mathbf{b})} = \left\{ \boldsymbol{\varepsilon}^{\mathrm{T}} \boldsymbol{\varepsilon} \right\} \tag{4.4}$$

where $\boldsymbol{\varepsilon} = \tilde{\mathbf{d}} - \boldsymbol{\Phi}\mathbf{b}$, $\boldsymbol{\Phi} = \left[\mathbf{P} + \gamma \mathbf{S} \tilde{\mathbf{I}} \right]$, and $\mathbf{d} \in \Re^{nm}$,

from (4.3) it follows that

$$\mathbf{J}_{(\mathbf{b})} = \left\{ \left(\tilde{\mathbf{d}} - \boldsymbol{\Phi}\mathbf{b} \right)^{\mathrm{T}} \left(\tilde{\mathbf{d}} - \boldsymbol{\Phi}\mathbf{b} \right) \right\} \tag{4.5}$$

In order to minimise the cost function $\mathbf{J}_{(\mathbf{b})}$ it is required that the partial derivatives of $\mathbf{J}_{(\mathbf{b})}$ with respect to the IMBs of **b** should be simultaneously zero. i.e.

$$\left. \frac{\delta \mathbf{J}_{(\mathbf{b})}}{\delta \mathbf{b}} \right|_{\mathbf{b} = \hat{\mathbf{b}}} = \mathbf{0} \tag{4.6}$$

where $\hat{\mathbf{b}}$ denotes the value of **b** which minimise (4.3)
Expanding (4.5) gives

$$\mathbf{J}_{(\mathbf{b})} = \mathbf{d}^{\mathrm{T}}\mathbf{d} - \mathbf{b}^{\mathrm{T}}\boldsymbol{\Phi}\mathbf{d} - \mathbf{d}^{\mathrm{T}}\boldsymbol{\Phi}^{\mathrm{T}}\mathbf{b} + \mathbf{b}^{\mathrm{T}}\boldsymbol{\Phi}^{\mathrm{T}}\boldsymbol{\Phi}\mathbf{b} \tag{4.7}$$

Making use of the vector differentiation [1, 117] leads to

$$\frac{\delta \mathbf{J}(\mathbf{b})}{\delta \mathbf{b}} = -2\boldsymbol{\Phi}^{\mathrm{T}}\mathbf{d} + \left(\boldsymbol{\Phi}^{\mathrm{T}}\boldsymbol{\Phi} \right)^{\mathrm{T}} \mathbf{b} + \left(\boldsymbol{\Phi}^{\mathrm{T}}\boldsymbol{\Phi} \right) \mathbf{b} \tag{4.8}$$

and since $\boldsymbol{\Phi}^{\mathrm{T}}\boldsymbol{\Phi}$ is a symmetric matrix it follows that:

$$\boldsymbol{\Phi}^{\mathrm{T}}\boldsymbol{\Phi} = \left(\boldsymbol{\Phi}^{\mathrm{T}}\boldsymbol{\Phi} \right)^{\mathrm{T}} \tag{4.9}$$

giving

$$\left. \frac{\delta \mathbf{J}_{(\mathbf{b})}}{\delta \mathbf{b}} \right|_{\mathbf{b} = \hat{\mathbf{b}}} = -2\boldsymbol{\Phi}^{\mathrm{T}}\tilde{\mathbf{d}} + 2\boldsymbol{\Phi}^{\mathrm{T}}\boldsymbol{\Phi}\hat{\mathbf{b}} \tag{4.10}$$

Equating to zero for a minimum yields

$$\mathbf{\Phi}^{\mathrm{T}}\tilde{\mathbf{d}} = \mathbf{\Phi}^{\mathrm{T}}\mathbf{\Phi}\hat{\mathbf{b}} \tag{4.11}$$

which leads to

$$\hat{\mathbf{b}} = \left[\mathbf{\Phi}^{\mathrm{T}}\mathbf{\Phi}\right]^{-1}\mathbf{\Phi}^{\mathrm{T}}\mathbf{d} \tag{4.12}$$

which is the optimal estimate of the IMBs in the sense of least squares.

Note that the above solution, which makes use of the so called pseudo inverse $[\mathbf{\Phi}^{\mathrm{T}}\,\mathbf{\Phi}]^{-1}\,\mathbf{\Phi}^{\mathrm{T}}$ [125], is only valid when a single beam is considered. Such an approach could be used to compensate for the presence of inhomogeneities (see Fig. 4.3) or non flat patient contours for a particular beam whilst making use of classical beam compensating techniques for the other beams involved in the treatment. Note that the patient contour correction, particularly in the head and neck region as well as the breast, is currently an area where active use is made of compensators [4], whereas the use of compensators to deliver intensity modulated beams is still very much in its infancy.

In order to illustrate the approach for a single beam, ILS has been used to compensate for the presence of inhomogeneities in order to produce a flat isodose profile at a depth of 10 cm (standard measurement depth for BSI and ICRU Report 50) [24, 64], see Fig. 4.3. Light grey areas correspond to regions of low density whilst dark grey areas correspond to regions of higher densities. Uncompensated, the dose delivered by the beam is higher in the inhomogeneity regions, due to the lower densities of the medium considered (see Chap. 2 and 3).

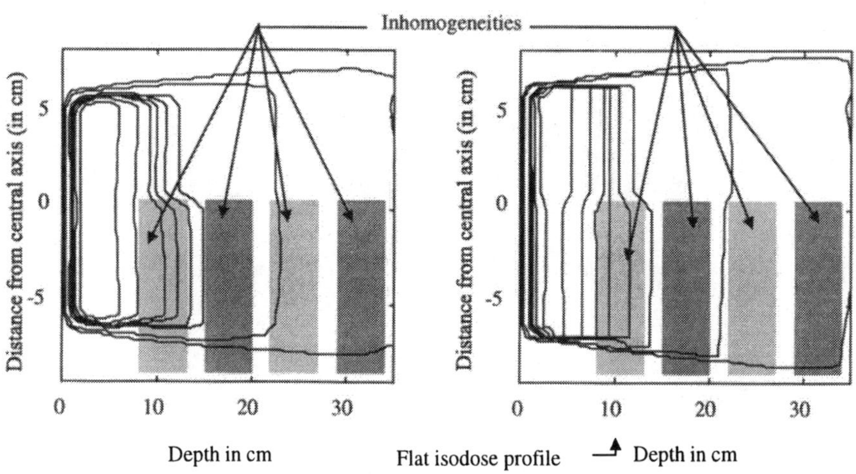

Fig. 4.3 Illustrating the use of the ILS algorithm to compensate for the presence of inhomogeneities for a single beam

It is shown in Fig. 4.3 that by increasing the dose in the upper half of the beam (left hand side from the beam's eye view), it is possible to produce a flat profile at the depth required. The resulting isodose plots optimised with use being made of a parallel beam have been mapped onto the profile of a divergent beam for display purposes.

This result provided the confidence to extend the approach to multiple beams. Indeed, RTP makes use of multiple fields [2, 3, 4], in which the task of providing the desired dose is shared among a number N_{beam} of beams. As a result, the solution of the inverse problem becomes an iterative process whereby the error is reduced at each iteration until the desired dose is achieved within some predefined tolerance bound.

4.3.2 Multiple Beam Formulation

In order to accommodate multiple beams, an iterative least square solution is required to be formulated. For each beam it is required to take into account different beam entry and gantry angle [28, 29, 30, 119, 126, 127] (see Chap. 5). The solution of the inverse problem for multiple beams can be seen as a pseudo parallel process. This process is illustrated in Fig. 4.4.

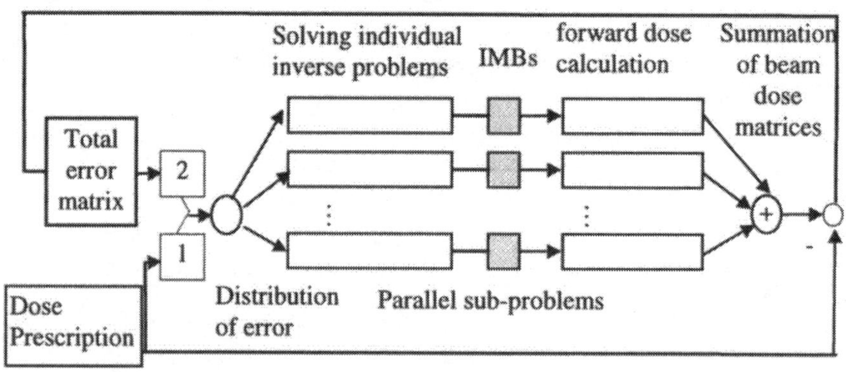

Fig. 4.4 Schematic representation of the iterative approach to the inverse problem

The initial stage involves the sharing of the dose prescription between the different beams in the system. Each individual beam sub-system is then solved semi-independently, to obtain a prescription specific set of IMBs for each sub-system. Following the first estimation of the values of the IMBs, each beam dose distribution is calculated and then combined to give the first estimate or prediction of the total dose. This dose is then compared with the dose prescription and an error is deduced. From this error a new estimate can be calculated to iteratively refine the solution. The distribution of the error and the summation stage of the beams involve a procedure detailed in [1] for parallel beams, with a flow chart comparing the summation/allocation procedure for parallel and divergent beams being given.

Summary of the Processes Involved in the Solution of the Inverse Problem for Multiple Beams. Exploiting the availability of parallel processing each sub-problem could be implemented on a different processor, with each processor performing tasks necessary to:

- extract the individual error allocated to each beam
- solve each inverse problem
- calculate the beam dose distribution
- rotate and map of the resulting dose distribution onto the reference grid

with the sequential processes being:

- the summation of all the dose distributions
- the comparison between prescribed and calculated total dose
- the allocation of a portion of the error to each sub-system.

Note that the pseudo parallel solution of the inverse problem has been implemented in a sequential manner in this work [119].

A purely sequential implementation has also been investigated in [108], where one set of IMBs is evaluated at each iteration. The approach has shown some interesting potential as less solutions of the pseudo inverse are required per iteration, with the number of iterations being of the same order of magnitude. However, the approach has been shown to be more sensitive to the apportionment of the error than the pseudo parallel scheme. Indeed, depending on the plan to be optimised, equal partitioning of the error may not be the best method.

In this work a traditional error allocation scheme has been adopted, where the error at each successive iteration is shared among the designated beams (i.e. if there are N_{beam} beams then each beam is required to deal with a portion of the error ε/N_{beam}.). This strategy is seen as appropriate because it guides the algorithm to a solution where all the beams contribute in an 'equal' manner to produce a well balanced plan, thus minimising the risk of creating hot spots [118, 119, 128] (see Chap. 5). A flow chart representation of the ILS algorithm is given in Fig. 4.5, where $\rho_i \in \aleph$ represents the apportionment of the error vector, here $\rho_i = N_{beam}$, $i = 1 \ldots N_{beam}$.

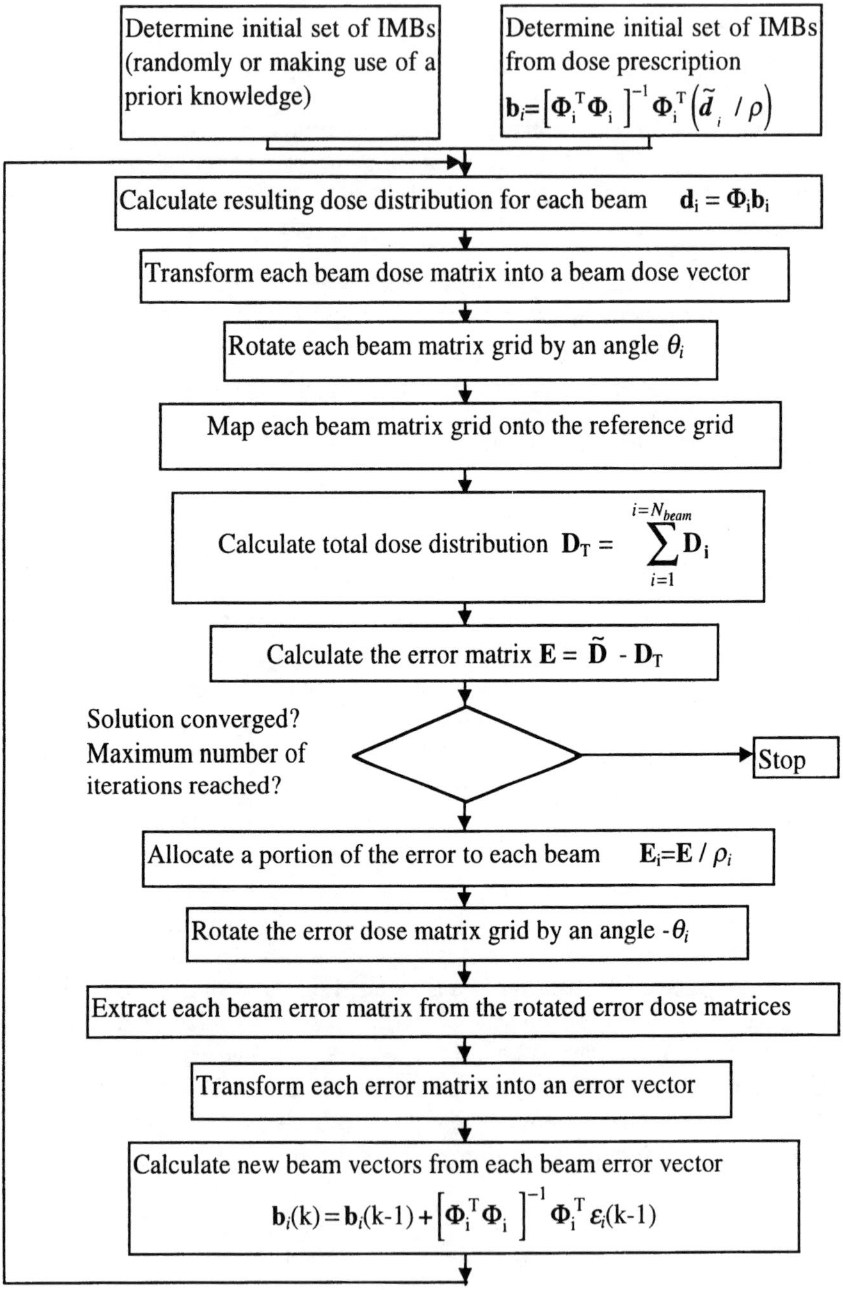

Fig. 4.5 Diagrammatic representation of the ILS procedure

Remark: The advantage of ILS over other gradient search techniques is that it is only necessary to calculate the matrix $[\mathbf{\Phi}^T\mathbf{\Phi}]^{-1}\mathbf{\Phi}^T$ once per beam, assuming that the position of the beam and/or the patient geometry does not vary during the course of the treatment. This is to be compared to the Newton method where the estimate of the Hessian is required to be calculated at each iteration.

4.3.3 Assessment of the ILS Algorithm on Standard Test Cases

In order to demonstrate the capabilities of the ILS scheme for multiples beams, the developed algorithm is tested on two standard test cases, namely a hinged pair and a three field brick with use being made of a 25 MV beam (see Chap. 2 and 3). The hinged pair and three field brick configurations are illustrated in Fig. 4.6 and 4.7 respectively.

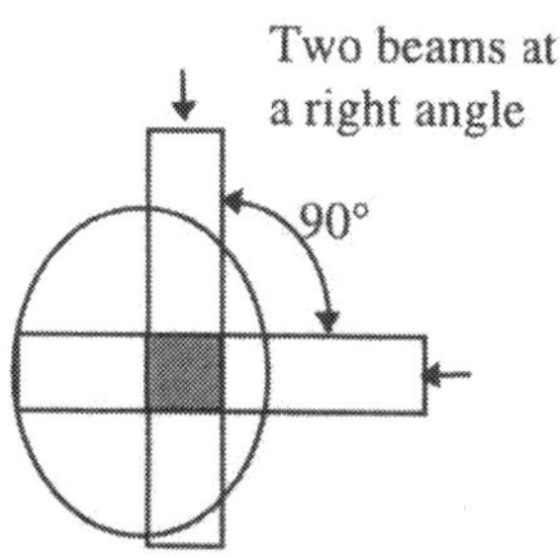

Fig. 4.6 Hinged pair used for head and neck cancer

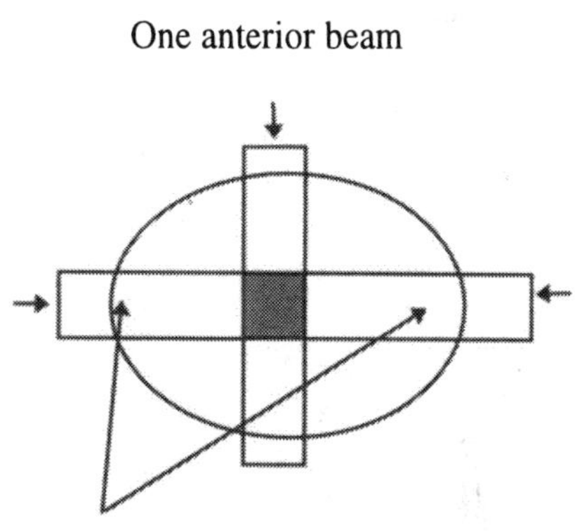

Fig. 4.7 Three field brick used for cancer in the pelvic region

Assessment of a Radiotherapy Treatment Plan. Methods for assessing a treatment plan rely traditionally only on visual inspection of the isodose plots. However, this method is limited to the 2-D case. In 3-D it is rather more difficult to appreciate the quality of the plan from visual inspection only. In order to facilitate a more quantitative assessment, dose volume histograms can be used. These relate the volumes of the various ROIs concerned to the dose received. In the work reported in this monograph, consideration is given to the 2-D case. Consequently, dose area histograms are employed. There are two categories of dose volume/area histograms:

- Integral or cumulative dose area/volume histograms [3, 4] give the area of the ROIs with respect to the %DD. Effectively it is the sum of the number of elements (dose grid points) receiving a dose higher or equal to a specific dose
- Differential dose area/volume histograms [3, 4] give the number of cells in the ROI receiving a certain amount of the dose. Dose area histograms used in this work assume a bin size of unity [3], i.e. grid point are considered to belong to the same bin if their dose lie in the predefined dose range. For example with a bin size of unity, dose increment of 1% are considered and the resulting intervals are [0% 1%), [1% 2%), ... [109% 110%], for dose levels between 0% and 110%.

The test cases together with subsequent treatment plans are assessed by making use of both visual inspection of the dose distributions and dose area histograms. The visual inspection provides qualitative information whereas the dose area histograms provide quantitative information.

Hinged Pair. The hinged pair involves the use of two beams at right angles as illustrated in Fig. 4.8 with wedge shaped compensators of opposite angle.

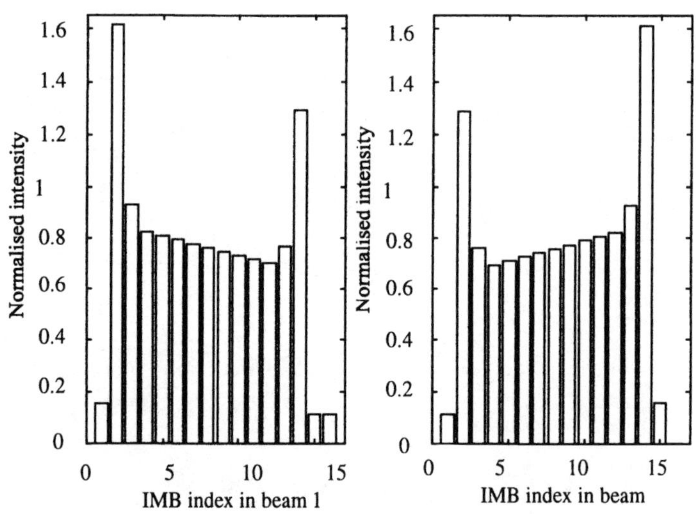

Fig. 4.8 Beam profiles for the hinged pair

The combination of the two beams can then produce a uniform dose for a square PTA. In this example, the hinged pair is used on a square shaped body contour of dimension 30 cm × 30 cm, with a square PTA of dimension 6 cm × 6 cm, such that the isocentre of the PTA corresponds to the isocentre of the idealised body contour. Note that the hinged pair would normally be used for head and neck cancer, with a body contour much smaller, therefore, than the one considered in this particular case. However, such a 'large' body contour helps in the visualisation of the outcome of the plan. The beams resulting from the optimisation are shown in Fig. 4.8 and the resulting isodose plot is shown in Fig. 4.9.

Note that large values of IMBs (>0.8) on the edge of each beam results from the compensation for the penumbra. In particular, it can be observed that IMBs with normalised values of 1.6 are twice the value they would have been, had the penumbra not affected the dose in the PTA. In practice the effect of the penumbra is non compensated, therefore, the selection of the field size allows for the presence of the penumbra, such that the sharp reduction of the dose on the beam edges occurs outside the PTA.

It is interesting to note that the wedge angles of the two beams are opposite with an absolute value close to 45°. This confirms that the optimisation algorithm is able to replicate the treatment planner's solution. Note the presence of unavoidable hot spots at the point of equilibrium (x_{max}) where the dose reaches 85%, with a large area receiving more than 70%. Note the rapid decay of the dose on the edge of the field.

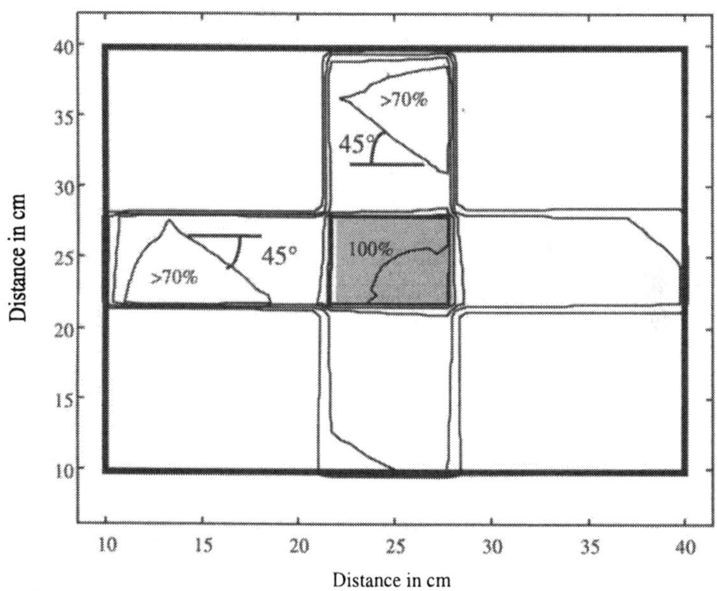

Fig. 4.9 Isodose plots for a hinged pair, the beams entering from the top and the left size

Figure 4.10 represents dose area histograms for the hinged pair. Note the rapid decay of the curve for the integral dose area histogram around a %DD equal to 100% for the PTA. Ideally one would require that the integral dose area histogram for the PTA to have a vertical edge at 100%, i.e. all the cells in the PTA receive at least 100% of the dose. The differential dose area histogram for the PTA is required to have single peak at 100%, which would mean that all the grid points in the PTA receive exactly 100% of the dose. The integral dose area histogram for the OHT should decay as fast as possible so that the number of cells receiving any dose is minimum. The differential dose area should have a very small number of cells receiving a high dose, i.e. above 60%. Figure 4.10 confirms the presence of hot spots, with a large number of grid points in the OHT receiving a %DD greater than 50%. It also confirms that the prescribed dose is achieved with good accuracy in the PTA.

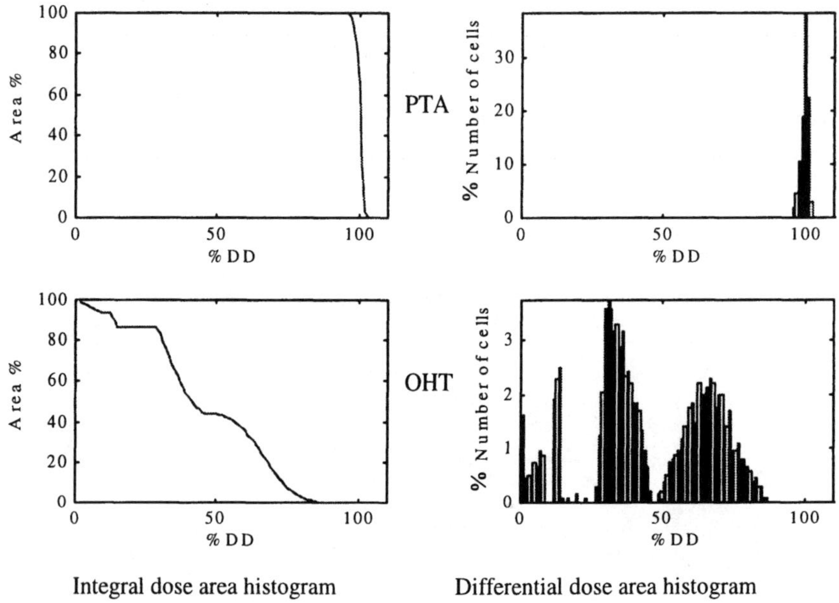

Fig. 4.10 Hinged pair - Integral (left) and differential (right) dose area histograms for the PTA (upper) and the OHT (lower)

Three Field Brick. The beam arrangement for the second test case is often used to deliver dose for cancer situated in the pelvic region. A three field brick involves three beams: one anterior beam and two parallel opposed beams as illustrated in Fig. 4.7. The anterior beam is usually an open field, whereas the parallel opposed beams make use of wedges which have opposite angles. The aim of the wedges is to compensate for the decay of the dose along the CAX of the anterior beam. The absence of wedges would create a higher dose in the upper part of the PTA if the parallel opposed beams were just open fields.

Again the IMBs optimised reproduce expected solutions (see Fig. 4.11). Note that beam 2 (the anterior beam) is slightly stronger that the parallel opposed beams. This results in the equalisation of the dose outside the PTA, thus avoiding unbalanced plans [108, 126, 128]. Again the high valued IMBs on the edge of the field, which attempt to compensate for the penumbra, are noted. In practice, however, it should be noted that it may be difficult to produce such IMBs.

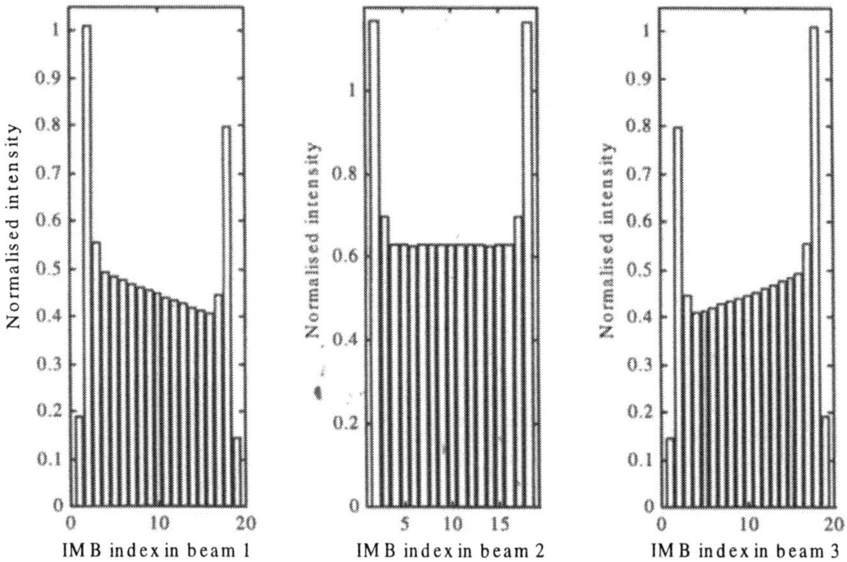

Fig. 4.11 IMB profiles for the three field brick (test case 2)

Figure 4.12 shows the resulting isodose plots for the three field brick. Note the symmetry of the plan with respect to the CAX of the anterior beam (vertical beam).

Figure 4.13 represents the dose area histograms for the three field brick. Note that all the grid points in the PTA receive a dose between 98% and 100%, with a small number of cells receiving a dose between 100% and 102%. Most of the cells in the OHT receive a dose below 65%. This indicates that the plan is well balanced, with the absence of any isolated spikes in the high dose region. The dose in the OAR, located in the beam path of the anterior beam is below 50%. This is a relatively high value and is due to the fact that the cost weighting coefficients chosen attach almost identical importance to the OAR as to the OHT.

Note the symmetry of the dose distribution with respect to the CAX of the anterior beam.

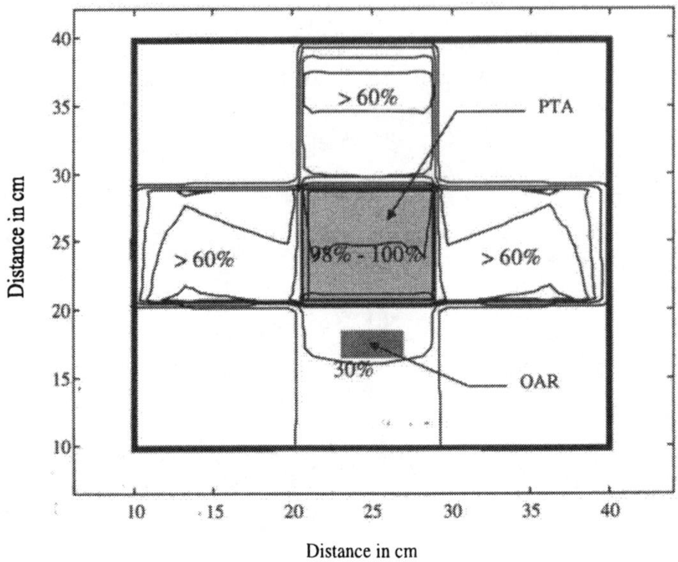

Fig. 4.12 Isodose plots for a three field brick

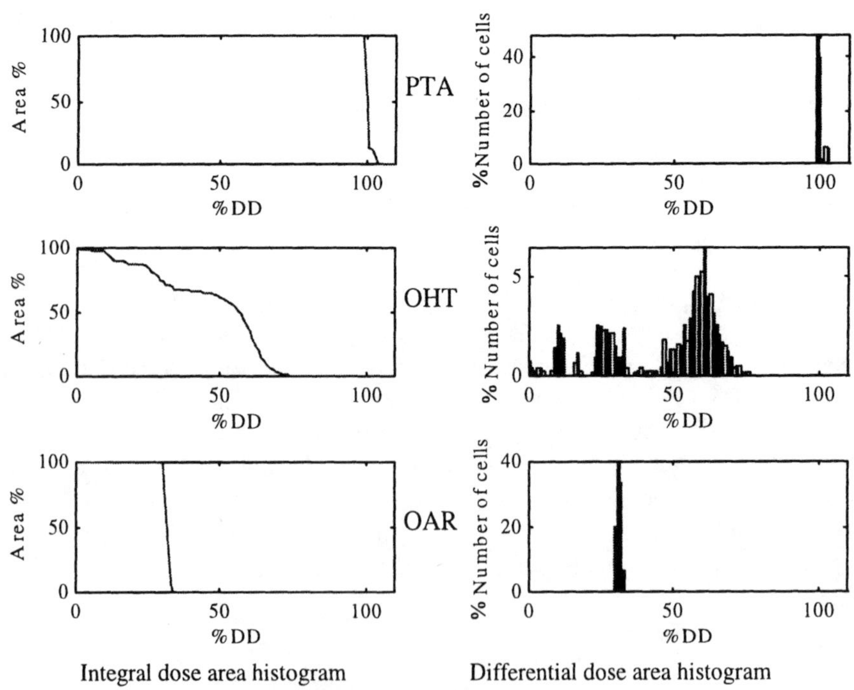

Fig. 4.13 Differential and integral dose area histograms for the three field brick

Remark: The results shown for the hinged pair and the three field brick involve the use of 25 MV beams. These are high energy beams compared to the 6 MV beams that are used in most centres to treat cancer in the pelvic region. Such high energy beams reduce the dose in the hot spots that can be observed at the points of equilibrium for each beam involved in the treatment. Indeed had a 6 MV beam been used for the hinged pair, hot spot as high as 115% would have been observed. This explains why plans in the pelvic region involve a minimum of three beams.

The hinged pair and the three field brick plans have helped to demonstrate that the ILS strategy combined with the parallel beam model can reproduce the prescription of the treatment planners. However, the aim of modulating the beam intensity is to attempt to conform to complex 'conformal prescriptions' involving concave PTA shapes. Such a plan involving a 'H' shaped PTA and two OARs is now used to highlight the full capabilities of the approach.

Conformal Prescription Plan with a 'H' Shaped PTA. The conformal test case involves a 'H' shaped PTA with two square OARs. The PTA is represented by a light grey area in Fig. 4.14, and the OARs by slightly darker square areas. This plan will be subsequently referred to as Plan 4.1. The treatment plan makes use of nine equispaced beams starting with a beam gantry angle at 90°. Although this plan is very unlikely to occur in reality, it is believed that it is perfectly suited to demonstrate the full capabilities of the optimisation algorithm to produce highly conformal treatment plans.

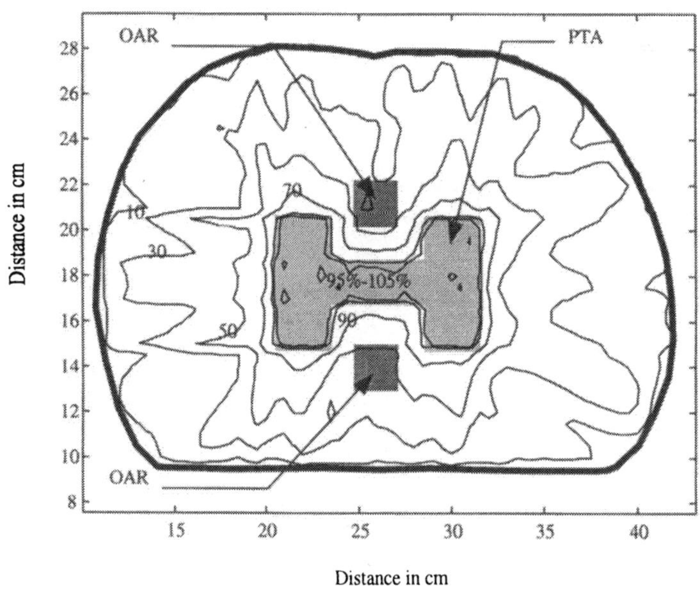

Fig. 4.14 Isodose plots of a treatment plan involving a H shaped PTA with two OARs

It can be observed in Fig. 4.14 that the isodose lines 90% and 95% conform almost exactly to the H shaped PTA, with most of the grid points in the PTA being between 95% and 105%, with a few hot spots at the intersection of the horizontal bar of the 'H' with its vertical bars (legs). This confirms findings from other workers [3] on 'H' shape like PTA.

Note that the dose at the corners of the 'H' shaped PTA is slightly below 90%. This is due to the fact that the optimisation algorithm is attempting to find a compromise between the OHT region, where the dose should be low and the PTA where the dose should be 100%. This can also be explained by the 'averaging' effect of the least squares cost function. This typical behaviour of ILS has prompted Lind [101] to argue that ILS was not suited for solving the RTP inverse problem as it may result in under-dosage in the PTA.

In order to counteract this effect, it may be necessary to emphasise the importance of the cells being on the edges of the PTA with respect to grid point in the remainder of the PTA. This can be achieved by allocating weightings to the different grid points that are considered in the optimisation (see Sect. 4.4). Alternatively it may be possible to artificially prescribe a higher dose to the grid points located at the edges. However, the test case used in this section is an extreme case, and it is believed that achieving only 95% on the edges will ensure that a lower dose is delivered to the surrounding healthy tissues.

The 50% isodose curve is shown to conform to the OARs. This is confirmed by the dose area histograms shown in Fig. 4.15. It can be observed, on the lower plots, that most of the cells in the OAR receive a dose less than 50% but all receive at least 30%.

Considering the dose area histograms concerning the OHT (middle plots of Fig. 4.15), it can be observed that most of the grid points receive a dose around 30%, which is the maximum dose prescribed. Note that no grid point in the OHT receives a dose above 85%.

The dose area histograms for the PTA (upper plots in Fig. 4.14) confirm the previous observations in that although most of the grid points receive a dose between 95% and 105%, few grid points receive less and a very small number receive more.

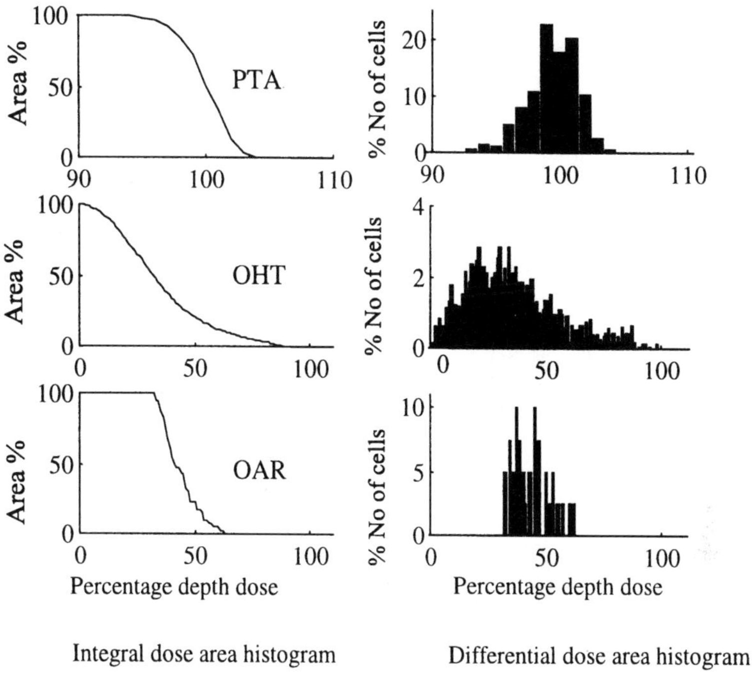

Fig. 4.15 Dose area histograms for a 'H' shaped PTA

Figure 4.16 shows the normalised intensities of the total IMB vector $\mathbf{b}_T$, defined such that:

$$\mathbf{b}_T = \begin{bmatrix} \mathbf{b}_1 \\ -- \\ \mathbf{b}_2 \\ -- \\ \vdots \\ -- \\ \mathbf{b}_{N_{beam}} \end{bmatrix} \quad (4.13)$$

where $\mathbf{b}_i$,i=1...N_{beam} are the IMB vectors for the individual beams involved in a plan. Note that the profiles of the beams are very irregular. In addition, the gradient between neighbouring IMBs in the same beam is large.

Remark: In Chap. 3 it has been argued that when use is made of patient specific compensators, only a limited gradient can be achieved. In fact, the results presented in this section can be considered as 'theoretical' results in the sense that they may not be physically or practicably achievable.

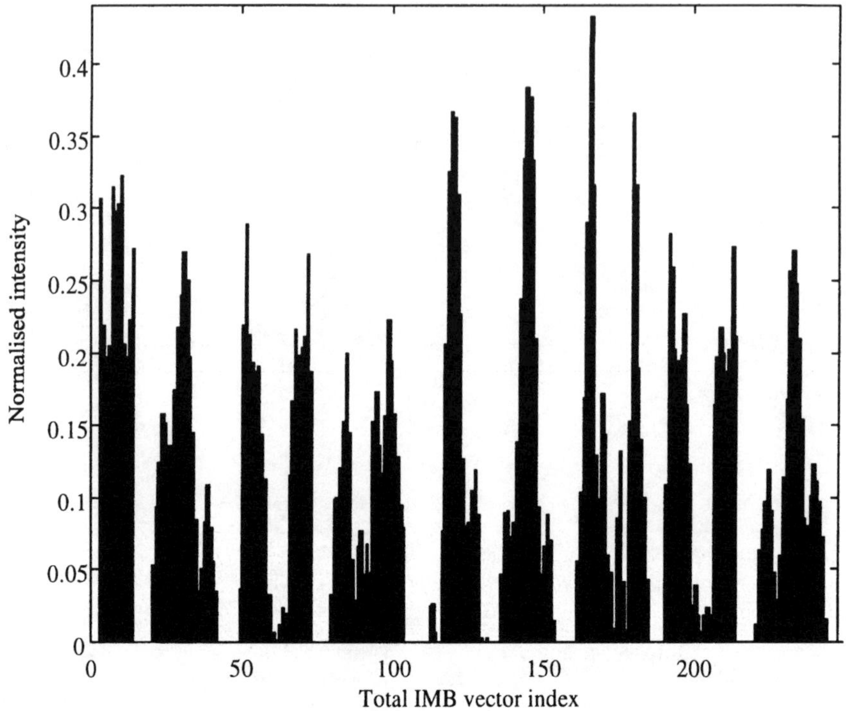

Fig. 4.16 Normalised intensity of the total IMB vector $\mathbf{b}_T$

Comparison Between a Conformal and Standard Treatment Plans. In order to highlight the potential benefits of intensity modulated radiation therapy, the 'H' shape conformal plan, i.e. Plan 4.1, making use of nine equispaced beams is compared to a four field brick (two pairs of parallel opposed beams). The four field brick is a technique favoured by several Hospitals, including the Christie Hospital in Manchester [34, 35]. The resulting dose distribution is shown in Fig. 4.17 and corresponding dose area histograms in Fig. 4.18. It can be observed that the dose in the PTA is achieved with good accuracy at the cost of an unacceptably high dose delivered to the OARs. Indeed some grid points in the OAR receive a dose as high as the dose received by the PTA. By comparison, the conformal plan delivers a dose in the PTA that is not as close to the ideal dose prescription, although, most of the dose grid points receive a dose that is within 5% of the dose prescribed. The main advantage of conformal radiotherapy is that the OARs may receive up to half the dose of the traditional four field brick. In addition, the presence of OARs in the anterior and posterior beam path leads to an unbalanced plan, where the dose in the OHT within paths of the left and right beams is much higher than the dose in the OHT in the paths of the other two parallel opposed beams. Indeed it is noted that although the dose within the PTA is homogeneous (between 99% and 102%), almost a quarter of the OARs receive an unacceptably high dose close to 100% with about 5% of the OHT receiving a similarly high dose.

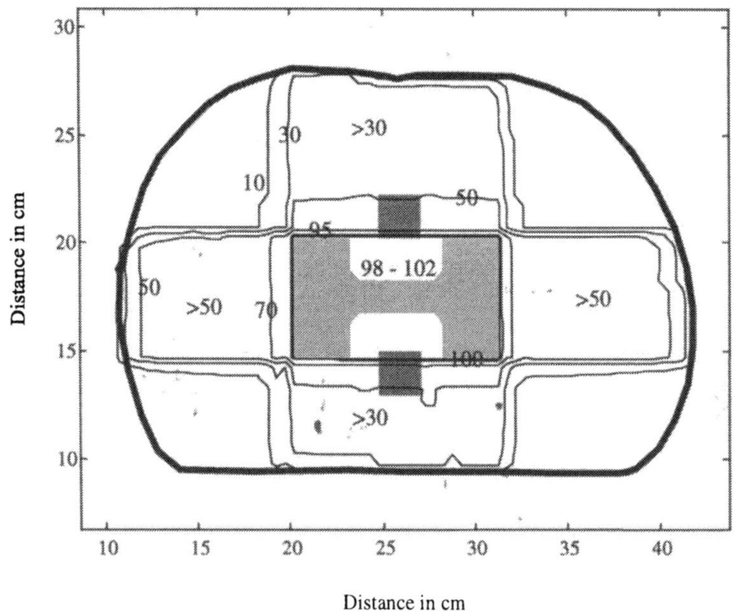

Fig. 4.17 Isodose contour plots for a 'H' shaped PTA treated with a traditional four field brick technique

Comparing the dose area histograms between the conformal plan (see Fig. 4.15) and the traditional plan (see Fig. 4.18), it can be observed that twice as many dose grid points in the OHT receive a dose greater than 50% when classical beam arrangement is used. Note, however, that when use is made of nine equispaced beams all the OHT receive some dose, whereas for a four field brick, some healthy tissues do not receive any dose radiation. This again shows that in RTP improvement in one area will most certainly lead to a degradation in at least one other area.

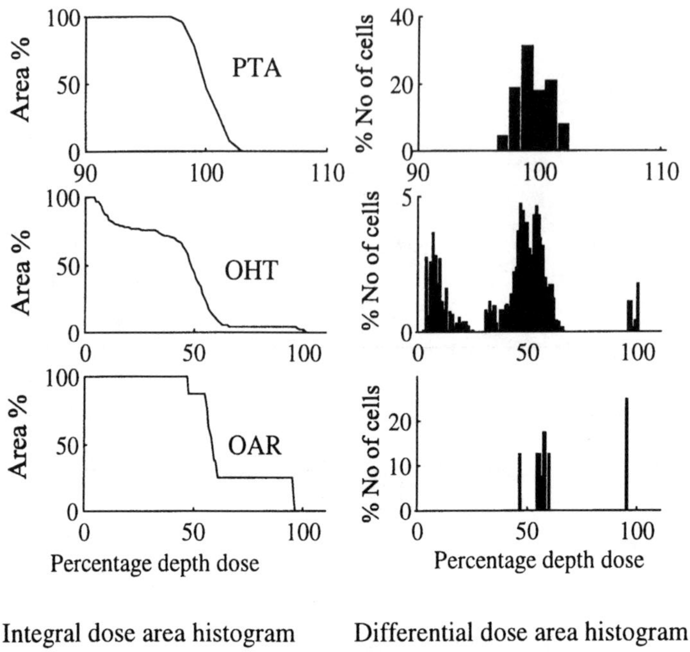

Fig. 4.18 Dose area histograms for a traditional four field brick

4.3.4 Introduction of Constraints on the IMBs

Non Negativity Constraint. Note that the solution of (4.12) may give rise to negative elements in **b**. However, once a dose of radiation has been delivered it is impossible to remove it. Therefore all the elements of **b** are required to be positive or null: $\mathbf{b} \geq \mathbf{0}$. This is traditionally achieved by a positivity operator that can be expressed under the following matrix form:

$$\text{diag}\mathbf{C} = \{c_{ii}\}, \text{ where } \begin{cases} c_{ii} = 1, b_i \geq 0 \\ c_{ii} = 0, b_i < 0 \end{cases} \tag{4.14}$$

Making use of such operator the iterative solution for a beam system is then as follows:

$$\mathbf{b}(k+1) = \mathbf{C}\left(\mathbf{b}(k) + \left[\mathbf{\Phi}^{\mathrm{T}}\mathbf{\Phi}\right]^{-1}\mathbf{\Phi}^{\mathrm{T}}\varepsilon\right) \tag{4.15}$$

However, such approach may not seem very rigorous mathematically. Another possibility to constrain the IMBs to be positive is to make use of cautious least squares.

Cautious Least Squares. It has been seen in Sect. 4.3.3 that a solution produced by the ILS scheme may not be physically achievable. This is due to the fact that the gradient between two neighbouring IMBs may not be physically reproducible. A new method which is introduced to constrain the gradient between neighbouring IMBs, is an approach derived from cautious least squares (CLS). CLS is activated if elements in the estimated IMB vector violate constraints on the allowable gradient of the IMBs. In this case, the IMBs violating the constraints are fixed to a value that satisfy the prerequisites on the allowable gradient. A new estimate of the IMB vector, with the IMBs violating the constraints kept constant is then determined.

In this case, CLS attempts to minimise the dual cost function

$$J_{CLS} = \left\| \tilde{d} - \Phi b \right\|^2 + \alpha \left\| \Delta b \right\|^2 \tag{4.16}$$

where the additional term involves minimising the gradient between neighbouring IMBs, with the scalar quantity $0 < \alpha$ chosen to emphasise the relative importance of the constraints imposed on the IMBs.

To illustrate this approach, use is made of CLS to determine the optimal combination of IMBs constrained to take the form of a wedge. The CLS scheme is tested on a plan previously shown in Fig. 1.8, and referred to as Plan 4.2 in this Chap. It corresponds to a prostate cancer patient referred to Walsgrave Hospital for treatment. It involves five fields selected using a method described in [28] and Chap. 5. The total IMB vector index optimised with both traditional and CLS approach is shown in Fig. 4.19.

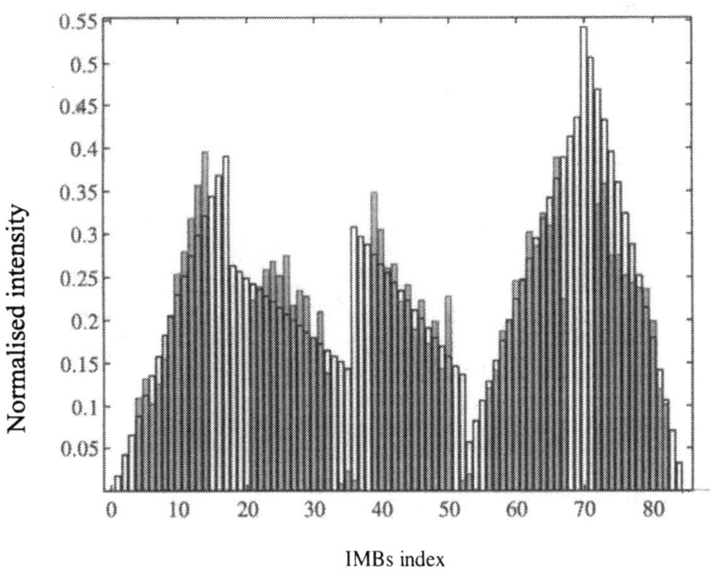

Fig. 4.19 Comparison between total IMB vector for constrained (unshaded) and unconstrained IMBs (shaded)

Figures 4.20 and 4.21 show the isodose contour plots displayed on the CT slice used to plan the treatment for the unconstrained ILS and the CLS scheme, respectively. The PTA is represented by dark grey area in the middle of the CT scan, see Fig. 4.20. The OARs, are the rectum and the spine and the femoral heads (see Chap. 1).

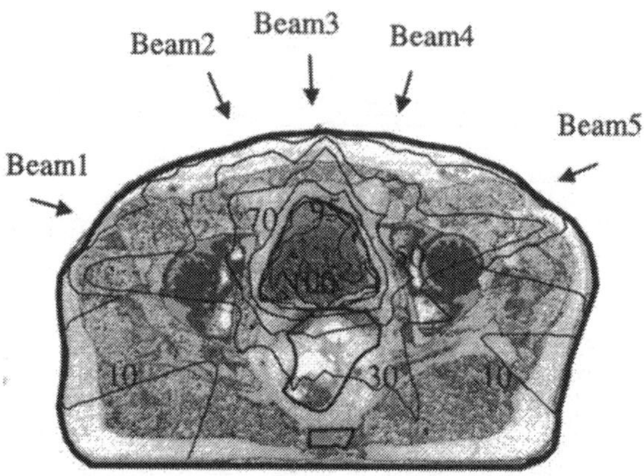

Fig. 4.20 Isodose contour plots for percentage depth dose of 100, 95, 90, 70, 50, 30 and 10 obtained for unconstrained IMBs

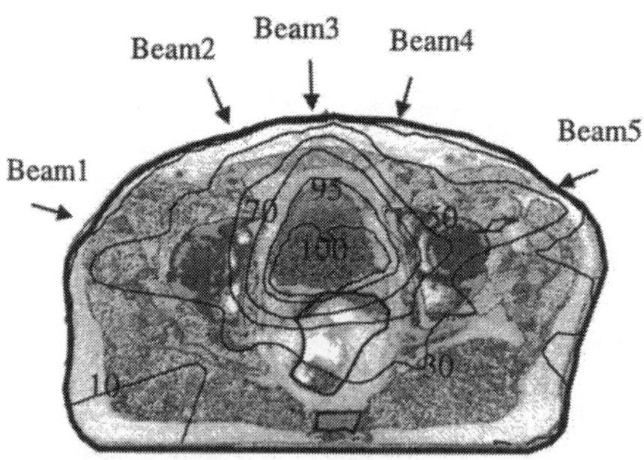

Fig. 4.21 Isodose contour plots for percentage depth dose of 100, 95, 90, 70, 50, 30 and 10 obtained for IMBs constrained to be wedged shaped beams

It can be observed that there is good agreement for the original beam profile and the constrained IMBs. Note however that the dose on the edges of each of the beam is much higher for constrained IMBs than for unconstrained IMBs due to the fact that the beams are constrained to be wedges. This results in an increase in the dose delivered to the OHTs on the edges of the PTA (see Fig. 4.20 and Fig. 4.21). Figure 4.20 shows isodose contour plots that conform very accurately to the PTA, whereas the isodose plot produced by the constrained beams, shown in Fig. 4.21, is characterised by much smoother contours. The latter is due to the fact that large changes in neighbouring IMBs that were enabling accurate conformation of the dose prescription have been reduced. This is also accompanied by a smoother and more uniform dose in the PTA when IMBs are constrained to smooth shapes. These findings are confirmed by the dose area histograms shown in Fig. 4.22. In particular it can be observed that all the ROI receive a smaller dose with the unconstrained IMBs. Constraining IMBs, including the edge of the fields result in a much higher dose in the OARs (black curve) with a few cells receiving up to 90% compared to a maximum dose of about 65% for the unconstrained IMBs (grey curve).

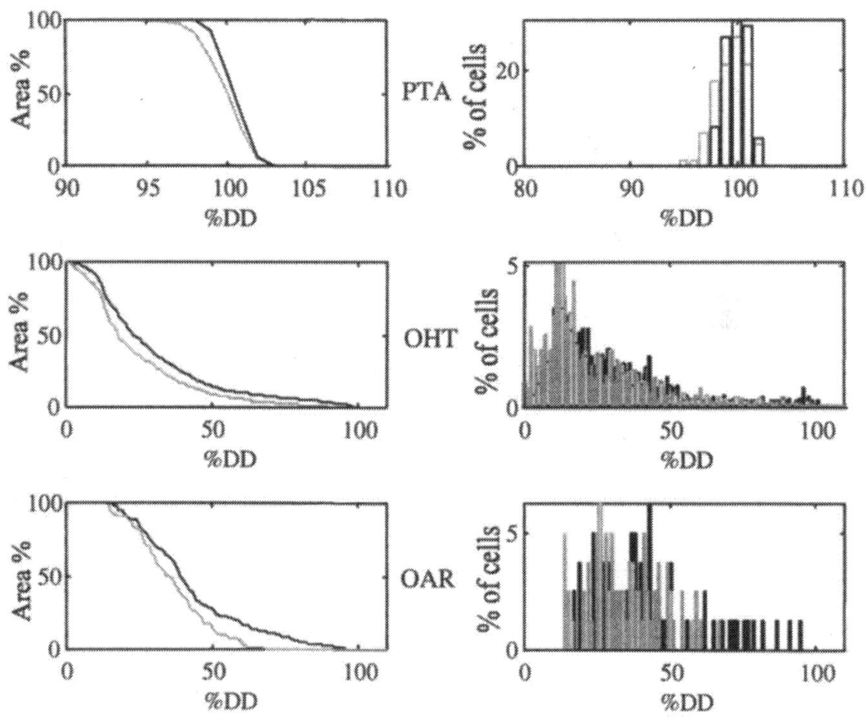

Fig. 4.22 Dose area histograms for Plan 4.2, unconstrained IMB (grey), constrained (black)

As a conclusion, constraining the IMBs to produce wedge shapes will result in a dose distribution that is slightly worse than with unconstrained IMBs. However the resulting solution will be easier and more practical to implement. The ultimate aim is to be able to predict a solution that is both accurate and easy to deliver. Further work is required in this area to identify accurately the limits imposed by the tools used to produce IMBs; limits that are likely to change with the beam modulator.

4.4 Articulation of the Objectives

Optimisation methods based on least squares (LS) attempt to minimise a cost function of the form (4.3). In data fitting problems, where LS is a very popular method, the aim is to obtain a function to approximate the data [119]. In these applications, LS considers each point as being equally important and attempts to find a trade off by minimising the sum of the squares of the errors. In RTP all the dose grid points are not equally important. Indeed it is more important to deliver the prescribed dose to the PTA and to minimise the dose to the OAR than it is to achieve a particularly low dose in the OHT. In practice, each IMB is subjected to competitive goals, that is to minimise the dose in the OHT or the OAR which requires the IMB to have a low intensity, whereas dose points in the PTA require IMBs to take a higher value. Therefore, it is necessary, to weight the relative importance of the various dose points considered to prevent the value of the IMBs from oscillating between solutions satisfying the various goals independently, thus attempting to achieve a trade off solution obtained by appropriate weighting of the objectives. The weighting schemes described in previous work assume constant objective weightings α, β and $\gamma \in \Re^{+}$. In this work such a traditional approach is compared with an adaptive scheme that adapts the original weightings so that when the error at the dose points satisfies a set of constraints the weights are reduced or set to zero whereas the weighting on critical dose points is increased in order to satisfy the prescription and produce an acceptable plan.

4.4.1 Weighted Sum of the Objectives

The cost function used within the ILS schemes is deduced from the general form given by equation (1.4), that is the sum of objectives of the form given in (4.3) such that:

$$\mathbf{J}_{(\mathbf{b})} = \alpha \sum \left(\tilde{d}_{PTA} - d_{PTA}\right)^2 + \beta \sum \left(\tilde{d}_{OAR} - d_{OAR}\right)^2 + \gamma \sum \left(\tilde{d}_{OHT} - d_{OHT}\right)^2 \quad (4.17)$$

which gives in vector form:

$$\mathbf{J}_{(\mathbf{b})} = \left\{ \alpha \left[\tilde{\mathbf{d}}_{PTA} - \mathbf{d}_{PTA} \right]^{\mathrm{T}} \left[\tilde{\mathbf{d}}_{PTA} - \mathbf{d}_{PTA} \right] + \beta \left[\tilde{\mathbf{d}}_{OAR} - \mathbf{d}_{OAR} \right]^{\mathrm{T}} \left[\tilde{\mathbf{d}}_{OAR} - \mathbf{d}_{OAR} \right] \right.$$
$$\left. + \gamma \left[\tilde{\mathbf{d}}_{OHT} - \mathbf{d}_{OHT} \right]^{\mathrm{T}} \left[\tilde{\mathbf{d}}_{OHT} - \mathbf{d}_{OHT} \right] \right\} \tag{4.18}$$

where $\tilde{\mathbf{d}}$ represents the prescribed dose and $\mathbf{d}$ the calculated (or predicted) dose for each of the ROI; with initially α, β, $\gamma \in \Re^+$ being the cost/objective weightings chosen traditionally such that $\alpha \cong \beta >> \gamma$ to ensure that a high dose, according to prescription, is delivered to the PTA whilst a minimum dose is given to the OAR and a low dose is delivered to the OHT [3, 4, 35, 108, 119, 129, 130]. In this monograph it is considered that the most important objective is to achieve the prescribed dose in the PTA, therefore, the objective weightings are chosen such that

$$\alpha \geq \beta >> \gamma \geq 0 \tag{4.19}$$

In [1, 129, 130] it has been found that the choice of the cost weighting factors greatly influences the optimal dose distribution resulting from the optimisation. The choice of these cost weighting factors is based on an empirical process that attempts to find a compromise between all the objectives. In order to produce the required dose in the PTA it is necessary to choose α to be sufficiently large. Choosing a large value for β will force the algorithm to reduce the dose delivered to the OAR. However it may also reduce the dose to the PTA and create an unbalanced plan; such plans being characterised by unbalanced loading of the beams. In the worse case, some of the beams may be almost switched off, to avoid irradiating OARs, whereas others may account for a very large contribution. In order to reduce this undesirable effect of creating hot spots [24, 129], it is beneficial to increase the weighting factor γ. Indeed a value of γ between 0.1 and 0.5 will ensure that the dose distribution in the OHT is 'even'. It also leads to a more rapid 'fall off' of the dose on the edge of the PTA [129, 130]. Conversely a low weighting on the OHT increases the possibility of hot spots but improves the resulting dose in the PTA and the OAR. However, choosing γ to be of the same order of magnitude as α may result in an undesirable reduction of the dose in the PTA.

Note that the order of magnitude of the cost weightings depends on the relative sizes of the ROIs and the number of matrix grid points encompassed in each case. This explains why the weighting in the PTA is traditionally chosen to be an order of magnitude greater than the weighting in the OHT (the PTA is usually small compared to the OHT). Although each treatment plan requires a specific combination of cost weighting factors, typical cost weighting values for α, β, and γ are given respectively by α=4, β=2, and γ=0.1.

For completeness, typical ranges for the cost weighting factors used during this research for various treatment plans is given in Table 4.1.

Table 4.1: Range of the cost weighting factors associated with each of the regions of interest

Region of interest	PTA	OAR	OHT
Range of cost weighting factors	$1 \le \alpha \le 7$	$0 \le \beta \le 7$	$0 \le \gamma \le 1$

Implementation of a Priori Weighting. Traditionally only one weighting factor is associated for each of the ROI [3, 4, 7, 68, 97, 98, 99, 104]. These weightings remain the same throughout the iterative phase, ensuring that the chosen trade-off solution is determined. Implementing these weightings involves the use of a diagonal matrix, such that (4.13) becomes:

$$\Delta \mathbf{b} = \left[\mathbf{\Phi}^{\mathrm{T}}\mathbf{\Phi}\right]^{-1}\mathbf{\Phi}^{\mathrm{T}}(\mathbf{W}\boldsymbol{\varepsilon}) \tag{4.20}$$

where $\boldsymbol{\varepsilon}$ is the error vector defined in equation (4.4). The diagonal matrix $\mathbf{W}$ is given by:

$$\mathrm{diag}\mathbf{W} = \{w_{ii}\},\ \text{where} \begin{cases} w_{ii} = \alpha, \text{ if } d_{ii} \in PTA \\ w_{ii} = \beta, \text{ if } d_{ii} \in OAR \\ w_{ii} = \gamma, \text{ if } d_{ii} \in OHT \end{cases} \tag{4.21}$$

Note that in practice, the diagonal form of $\mathbf{W}$ is exploited in order to reduce the storage and computation requirements and use is made of a dot product of diag$\mathbf{W}$ with the error vector $\boldsymbol{\varepsilon}$.

In order to validate the approach of making use of *a priori* weighting, the scheme is tested on Plan 4.2, see Fig. 4.23. The resulting dose distribution displayed on the CT slice used to plan the treatment is shown in Fig. 4.23.

Note that the actual CT numbers are not used directly to calculate the dose distribution. Instead, inhomogeneous regions are outlined manually, with each region being associated with an attenuation coefficient (see Chap. 3). The influence of these inhomogeneities will be discussed later in Sect. 4.5.3.

Making use of fixed objective weightings, the ILS scheme is able to deliver a conformal irradiation to the prostate whilst sparing the spine and the rectum. In particular it can be observed that all the PTA receives between 95% and 105% whilst the rectum receives around 20% and the spine is completely spared. Note that the beam orientation has been optimised such that it spares the spine whilst ensuring a reasonable conformation of the PTA (see Chap. 5). Note that other beam arrangements could have been chosen to improve the degree to which the beams conform to the PTA, however this could have led to the irradiation of the spine.

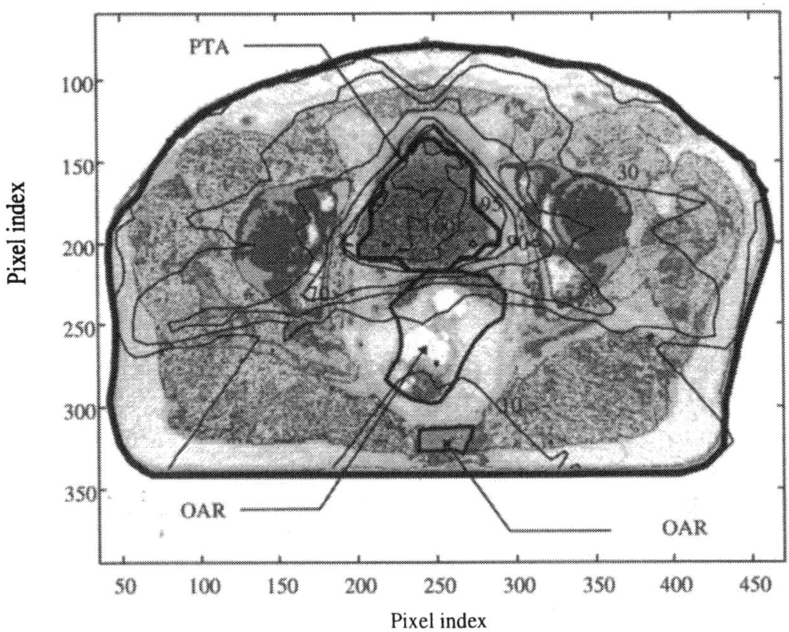

Fig. 4.23 Isodose contour plot for plan 4.2 optimised with ILS and fixed objective weightings

4.4.2 Adaptive Objective Weighting

The aim of the new adaptive weightings scheme proposed here is to focus the attention of the optimisation process on specific dose points that do not comply with acceptability criteria whilst, at the same time, disregarding dose points that are already considered as acceptable. As opposed to the previous scheme with fixed objectives, the adaptive weighting does not attempt to determine an optimal plan, but rather to solve for a set of IMBs that produce a plan within specification [130]. This scheme is believed to be beneficial to demanding treatment plans, where the dose prescription at some point may not be achievable. Under such circumstances, the aim is to attempt to find the closest achievable compromise.

The weighting scheme can also be viewed as that of making use of relaxation parameters to relax constraints on some of the regions whilst emphasising the relative importance of other regions that are required to be within specification at all cost. Table 4.2 presents a comparison between ideal dose, prescribed dose and acceptable doses in the various ROIs.

Table 4.2 Comparison between ideal prescribed and acceptable doses for PTA, OAR and OHT

ROI considered	PTA	OAR	OHT
Ideal dose in %	$d_{PTA} = 100$	$d_{OAR} = 0$	$d_{OHT} = 0$
Prescribed dose in %	$d_{PTA} = 100$	$d_{OAR} \leq 30$	$d_{OHT} \leq 40$
Acceptable dose in %	$95 \leq d_{PTA} \leq 105$	if possible $d_{OAR} \leq 30$	if possible $d_{OHT} \leq 40$

Prescribed Dose. In order to accommodate the prescription for the OAR and the OHT that are given in terms of an inequality, it is necessary to artificially alter the error, i.e. the difference between the dose prescription and the predicted dose. Indeed assuming that a prescription is implemented with use being made of (4.17), with d_{PTA} =100, d_{OAR}= 30, d_{OHT}=40, minimising the overall weighted sum may result in a plan which doses are higher than necessary. For example, ILS may attempt to achieve 40% dose in the OHT even when the dose is only 20%. Therefore for prescriptions given in terms of inequality, if the objective is satisfied at a particular grid point, then the error associated with this grid point is automatically set to zero such that (4.21) becomes:

$$\text{diag}\mathbf{W} = \{w_{ii}\} = \begin{cases} \text{if}(d_{ii} > \tilde{d}_{ii}), \begin{cases} w_{ii} = \alpha, ii \in PTA \\ w_{ii} = \beta, ii \in OAR \\ w_{ii} = \gamma, ii \in OHT \end{cases} \\ \text{else } w_{ii} = 0 \end{cases} \tag{4.22}$$

Setting the objective weightings to zero can be viewed in a similar manner to a controller with dead band, i.e. when the output is within some specified range, no action is taken. Similarly, in RTP, when the dose is within specification, the error associated with it is artificially reduced or set to zero so that it cannot influence the IMBs.

Extending this scheme to other dose levels is similar to designing an evolutionary decision maker (DM) that can adapt the weights of the objectives according to the dose value of each individual grid point.

In this case w_{ij} can be expressed as follows:

$$w_{ij} \begin{cases} i = j, w_{ij} = \alpha_{\text{ROI}} \text{DM}(d_{ij}, \text{ROI}) \\ w_{ij} = 0 \end{cases} \tag{4.23}$$

where d_{ij} are the dose values corresponding to matrix grid points, ROI is the region to which the grid point belongs (i.e. PTA, OAR or OHT), and DM(d_{ij}, ROI) represents the output of the decision maker that is function of the dose level at the point considered and of the type of ROI that the point belongs, and α_{ROI} (i.e. α, β and γ) are the a priori error weightings associated with the ROI considered. The aim of the DM is to modify the initial weightings of the objectives in order to adapt it according to the dose variation between grid points belonging to the same ROI. The procedure may be regarded as a primitive form of evolutionary scheme [119, 130].

In order to demonstrate the possible benefits of adapting the weighting to individual dose grid points the following DM has been designed such that the emphasis to dose grid points in the PTA within prescription is reduced whilst the emphasis to points in the OHT and OARs is increased. Fig. 4.24 shows the output of the DM, where DM(d_{ij}, ROI) = 1.0 represents the initial setting of the objective weighting factors.

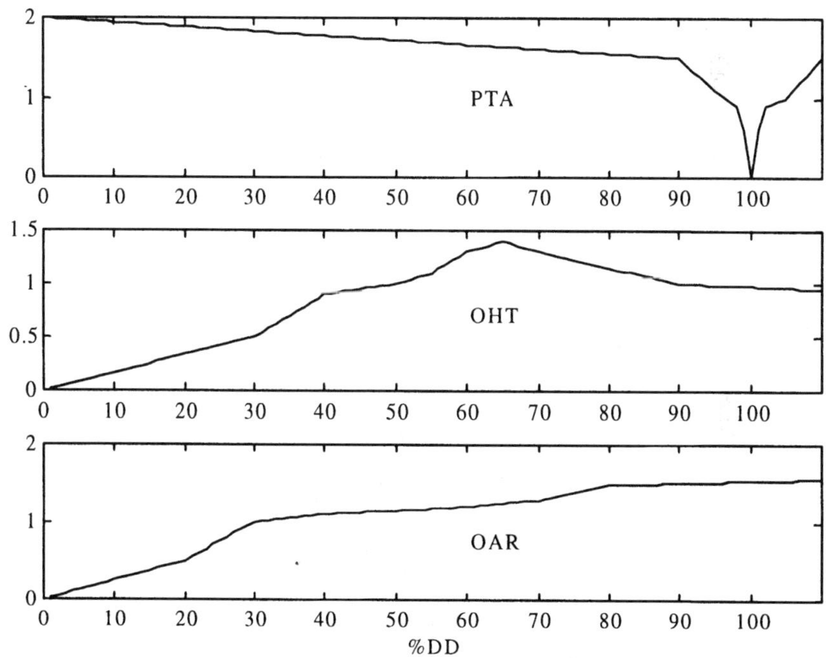

Fig. 4.24 Output of the decision maker when subject to a dose input varying between 0% and 110%, the upper Fig. showing the output of the DM for the PTA, DM(α, PTA), the middle Fig. the output of the DM for the OHT, DM(γ, OHT), and the lower Fig. the output of the DM for the OAR, DM(β, OAR)

Common to all the ROIs, is the 'dead band' like action, i.e. provided that a dose is within specification, its error is modified, i.e. set to zero or to a lower value, however as opposed to the 'pure' dead band, the error is not set to zero if it is within specification.

In order to emphasise the importance of achieving the dose prescription within 5 % in the PTA, weights associated with dose grid points belonging to the PTA are artificially increased for grid points receiving a dose greater than 102% or less than 98%. (see Fig. 4.24, upper). Reversibly, when the dose is within these bounds, the individual objective weightings (IOW) are set to a lower value.

Similarly, in the OAR, dose within prescription are associated with lower IOW values. However in order to minimise the maximum dose received by the OARs, the original objective weightings are increased as the dose received by the OAR increases (see Fig. 4.24, lower).

The same approach is adopted for the OHT, except that the relative increase with respect to the weightings associated with the OHT is rather more moderate (see Fig. 4.24, middle).

In order to assess the benefits of an individual weighting of the error associated to each dose grid point, Plan 1 is considered.

Comparison Between a Priori and Adaptive Weighting on Plan 4.1. Figures 4.25 and 4.26 show the isodose distribution resulting from the use of ILS with fixed objective weightings (FOW) and individual objective weighting (IOW), respectively. The resulting dose area histograms are given in Fig. 4.26.

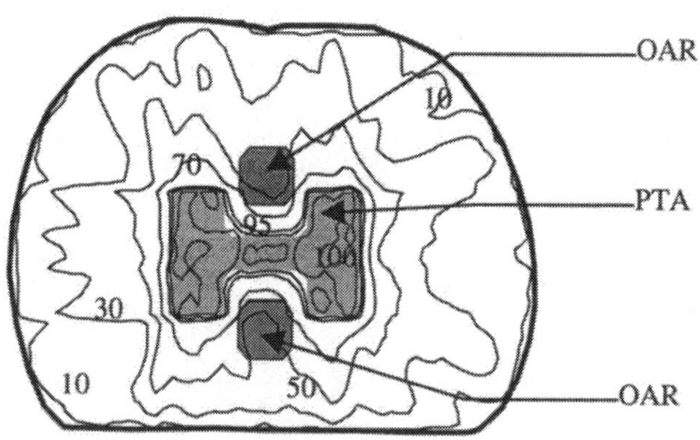

Fig. 4.25 Dose distribution obtained after 58 iterations using ILS with fixed weightings for Plan 4.1

It can be observed from Fig. 4.25 and 4.26 that the dose within the PTA is more homogeneous with FOW (more cells receive a dose close to 100%), whereas the dose received by the OAR is slightly reduced with the IOW scheme. However, in order to determine more precisely the effect of the IOW scheme it is necessary to make use of the dose area histograms represented in Fig. 4.27. It can be observed in Fig. 4.27a that more cells receive a dose between 98% and 102% for FOW, however a few cells receive a dose under that prescribed (i.e. under 95%). Making use of IOW reduces the weightings associated with the dose grid points within the PTA, leading to an increase in the number of cells receiving a dose between 95% and 99% and an increase in the number of cells receiving a dose between 102% and 105%. The main advantage of the IOW is that it forces all the points located in the PTA receive a dose within +/- 5% of that prescribed. In addition, the mean and the maximum dose received by the OARs are lowered, see Fig. 4.27b with IOW at no extra cost for the OHT, see Fig. 4.27c. Indeed, the dose area histogram for the OHT show no noticeable difference between the various schemes.

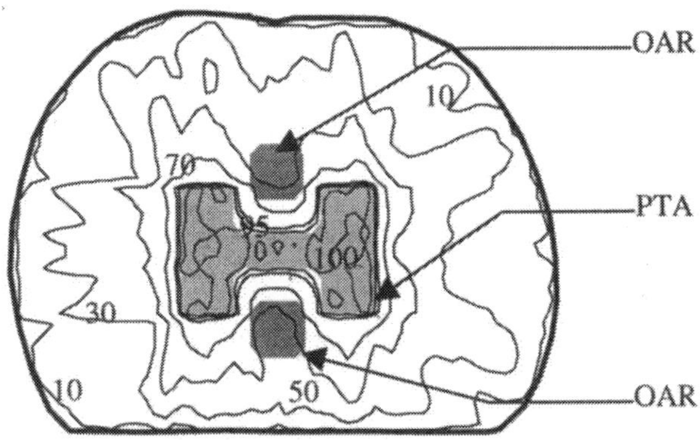

Fig. 4.26 Isodose contour plot obtained after 63 iterations using ILS with adaptive weightings for Plan 4.1

Remarks: Although the adaptive weighting scheme has been applied by considering the grid point dose levels together with their association to the ROI, it is possible to extend the scheme to account for the position of each point, thus ensuring that a dose at a particular point is exactly the specified value. This could prove particularly useful in ensuring that the dose on the edges of the PTA is high enough or that a specific OAR dose not receive more that its maximum allowable dose.

The output level of the DM should not be too high as it may cause the optimisation to oscillate between two goals that cannot be simultaneously achieved. When this occurs, it is possible with the DM to include information regarding the rate of change of the error, so that if the error oscillates or increases, the demands on the variable weighting factors associated with each ROI can be reduced or relaxed by reducing the values of some or all the cost weighting factors.

Determining an appropriate trade-off without *a priori* knowledge of the type of treatment plan is difficult and may become a lengthy process if all the objectives are competing with each other. However, in order to determine the relationships between the various objectives it is possible to use an alternative method which is based on the concept of Pareto optimality [11, 85]. This method, which is detailed in Chap. 5, enables the determination of an overall view of the relationships between the various objectives.

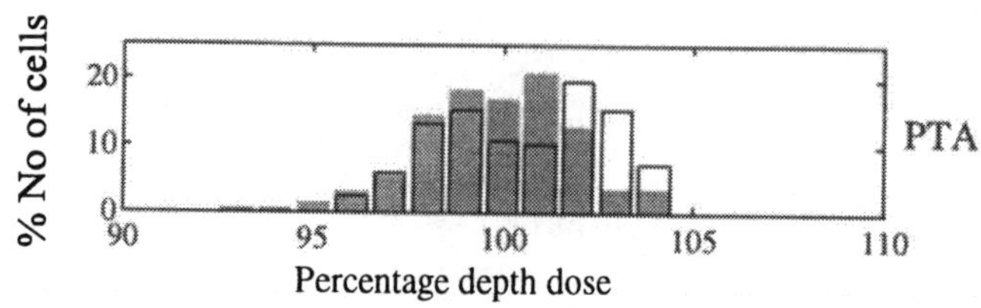

a) Differential dose area histograms of the PTA with IOW (unshaded) and fixed objective weightings (shaded)

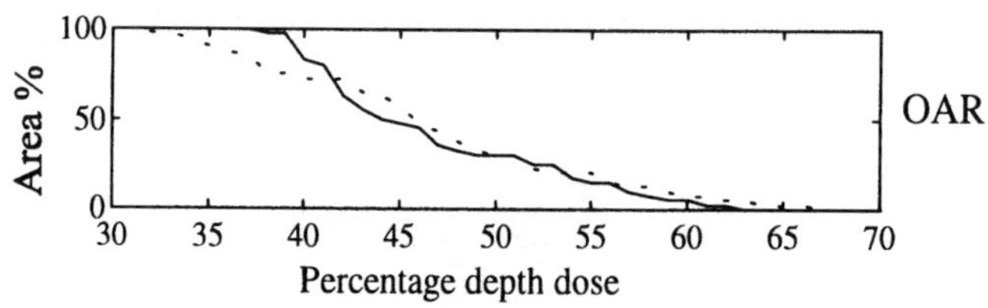

b) Integral dose area histograms of the OAR with IOW (plain) and fixed objective weightings (dashed)

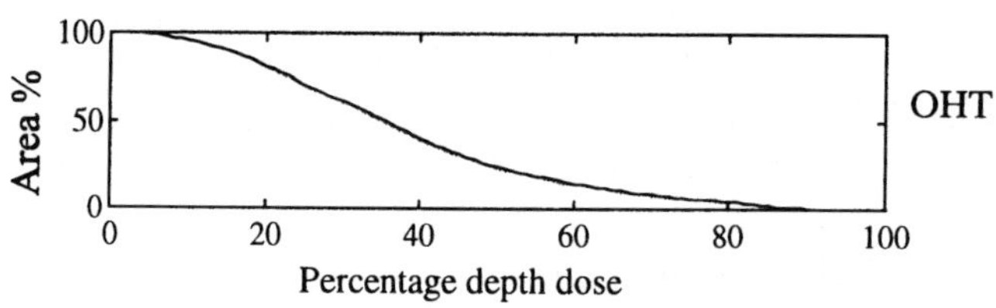

c) Integral dose area histograms for the OHT with IOW (black) and fixed objective weightings (grey)

Fig. 4.27 Illustrating the benefits of adaptive weighting over a priori weighting for plan 4.1

4.5 Improving the Rate of Convergence of the Algorithm

In previous work [68, 72, 80, 101], it has been shown that the use of scaling factors to multiply the information matrix or the Hessian matrix for optimisation methods based on ILS and gradient descent respectively can improve the convergence of the algorithm. This scaling factor increases the rate or speed of convergence of the algorithm by increasing the elemental step size, i.e. the amount of corrective action, from one iteration to the next. Further, it has been observed that in many cases approximations of Hessian matrices are used in the algorithm. Although this is not required in the ILS scheme adopted, the information matrix $\mathbf{\Phi}^T\mathbf{\Phi}$ being invertible. This section proposes various schemes combining the use of scaling factors to various modifications of the information matrix to determine their effects on the rate of convergence. Methods adopted are similar to those used in system identification e.g. forgetting factors and Kalman filtering.

In order to increase the rate of convergence of the ILS scheme, it is possible to decrease/inflate all the elements of the information matrix/inverse of the information matrix (i.e. the covariance matrix). This can be achieved by introducing a factor $\lambda \leq 1.0$ such that the information matrix becomes:

$$\mathbf{F}= \lambda\mathbf{\Phi}^T\mathbf{\Phi} \tag{4.24}$$

where $\mathbf{F}\in \Re^{n\times n}$ is referred to in this work as the modified information matrix. The effect of λ can be visualised in Fig. 4.28, where a reduction in the value of λ leads to an increase in the speed of convergence combined with a small reduction in the sum of the square of the weighted error.

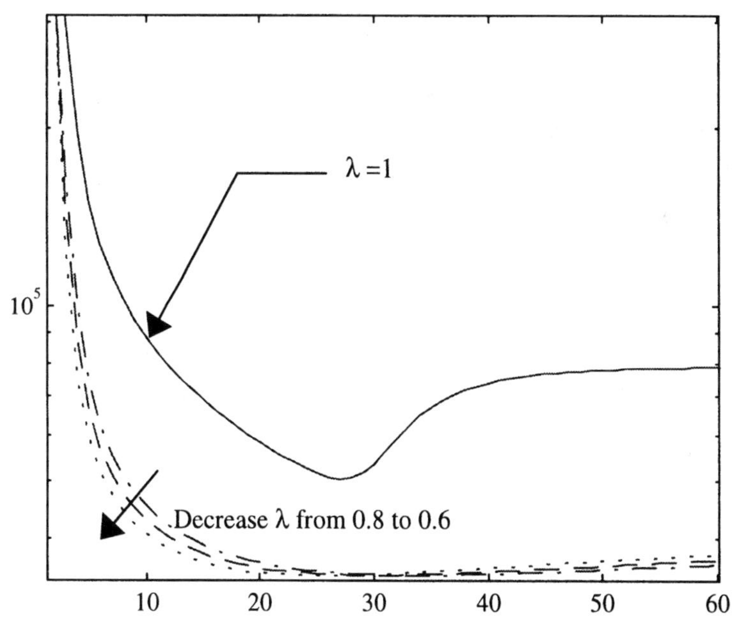

Fig. 4.28 Influence of the scalar λ in equation (4.24) on the rate of convergence

By adopting procedures of control theory, the introduction of the scalar λ to increase the rate of convergence is similar to the use of a forgetting factor in the recursive least squares (RLS) algorithm. Indeed a forgetting factor can be used to allow the estimated parameters of a control system to adapt more quickly to any change in the system by inflating the covariance matrix (inverse of the information matrix). The inclusion of forgetting factor has proven successful in control applications, however its performance may be impeded in the presence of noise and correlation between the elements of the covariance matrix. In order improve the situation techniques similar to these used in Kalman filtering (KF) can be used. The main difference between RLS with a forgetting factor and a KF used for estimation purposes is that in the KF the process noise covariance matrix $\mathbf{R}_w$ [124] is used to inflate only selected elements of the covariance matrix, thus providing an increased flexibility and selectivity. $\mathbf{R}_w$ is normally a diagonal matrix, so KF techniques can be seen as increasing the diagonal elements of the covariance matrix, which is similar to reducing the diagonal elements of the information matrix. Making use of the above observation, consideration is given to an alternative expression for the modified information matrix, given by

$$\mathbf{F} = \mathbf{\Phi}^T\mathbf{\Phi} - \lambda\,\mathrm{diag}(\mathbf{\Phi}^T\mathbf{\Phi}) \tag{4.25}$$

where $\lambda \in \Re^+$, with $0 \leq \lambda < 1$ to ensure that $\mathbf{F}$ remains positive definite. In this work the value of λ is taken in the range $0 \leq \lambda \leq 0.8$.

The influence of λ on the rate of convergence is illustrated in Fig. 4.29. It can be observed that a reduction of the diagonal elements leads to improvements in terms of both rate of convergence and reduction in error.

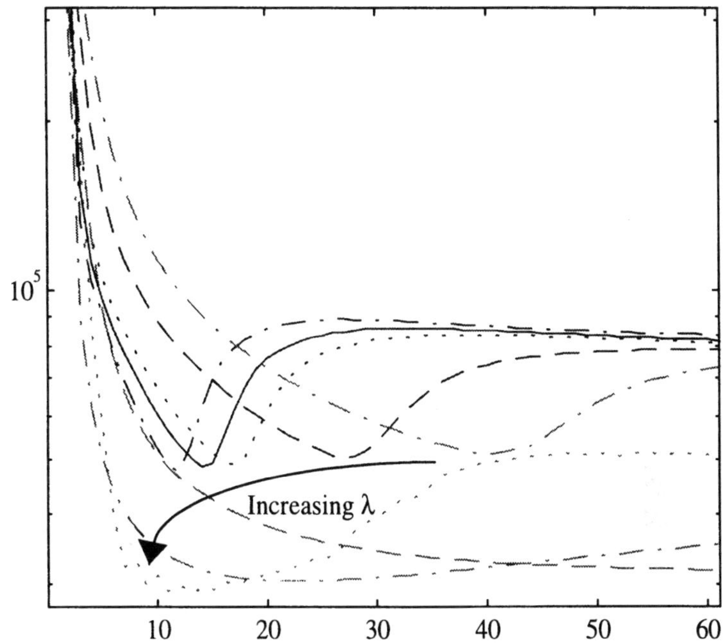

Fig. 4.29 Influence of the scalar λ in equation (4.5) on the rate of convergence

In gradient descent search techniques applied to RTP, the Hessian matrix is often taken as an identity matrix. Similarly in this work, the modified information matrix is approximated by the following expression:

$$\mathbf{F} = \lambda^{-1}\mathbf{I} \tag{4.26}$$

where $\lambda \in \Re^{+}$, $\lambda >> 0$.

The influence of λ is illustrated in Fig. 4.30. Once again it can be observed that a reduction in λ causes the algorithm to converge more rapidly to a better solution.

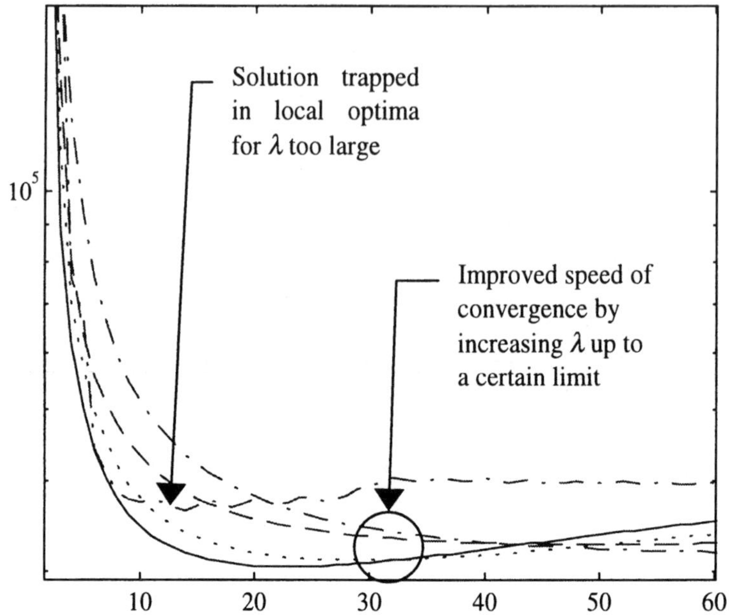

Fig. 4.30 Influence of the scalar λ in equation (4.26) on the rate of convergence

Finally, the last modification to the information matrix reported in this work is given by:

$$\mathbf{F} = \lambda \, \mathrm{diag}(\mathbf{\Phi}^T\mathbf{\Phi}) \tag{4.27}$$

The influence of λ is illustrated in Fig. 4.31. Once again it can be observed that a reduction in λ causes the algorithm to converge more rapidly to a better solution.

Adopting the above notation, the iterative step leading to the determination of each IMB vector **b** involved in a plan can be expressed as follows:

$$\mathbf{b}_k = \mathbf{b}_{k-1} + \mathbf{F}^{-1}\,\mathbf{\Phi}^T\,\mathbf{e}_k \tag{4.28}$$

where $\mathbf{b}_k$ is the IMB vector at the kth iteration, **F** is the modified information matrix, $\mathbf{\Phi}$ is the beam dose calculation matrix and $\mathbf{e}_k$ is the error at the kth iterations.

In order to compare the most appropriate approach to the solution of the inverse problem, the best solution obtained with each of the schemes is recorded in Fig. 4.32. It can be observed that reducing the values of the elements on the diagonal of the information matrix results in an improvement in the error compared to decreasing all the elements of the information matrix. The fastest convergence corresponding to a rapid reduction in error is obtained by making use of equation (4.25) [130].

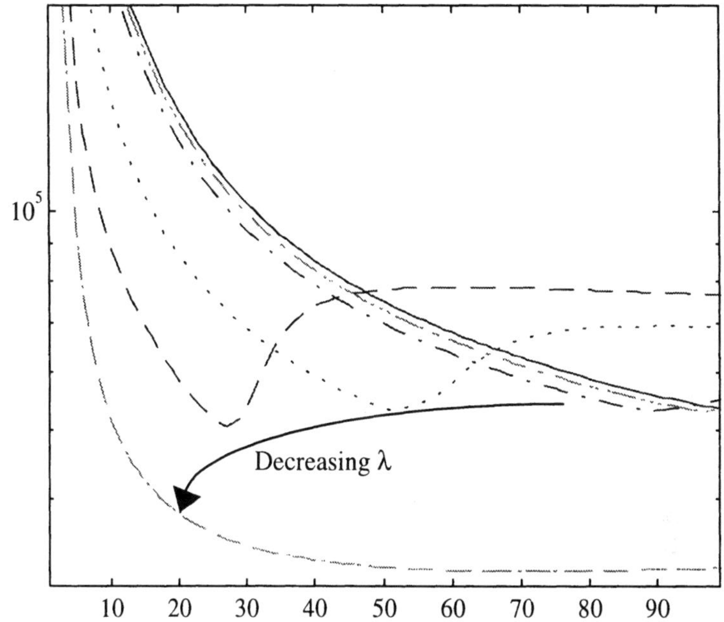

Fig. 4.31 Influence of the scalar λ in equation (4.27) on the rate of convergence

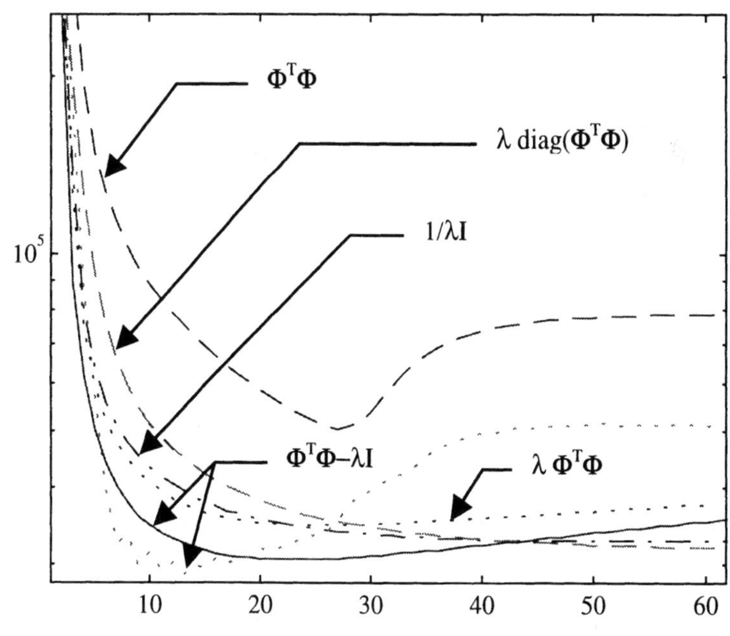

Fig. 4.32 Comparison between the various expression adopted for the modified information matrix

4.6 Simulation Studies

The aim of the simulation studies is to determine typical characteristics and behaviour of the ILS schemes. In particular, interest is focused on the influence of initial conditions and inhomogeneities.

4.6.1 Influence of the Initial Conditions

The aim of this section is to justify the approach adopted in this work which deduces an initial estimate of IMBs from the dose prescription. This initial beam setting is then iteratively refined using the scheme represented in Fig. 4.5. Several strategies exist to initialise the iterative algorithm.

A common approach to heuristic search [10] is to set the IMB to a random value. However, such a random initialisation, in the presence of concave PTA, may result in the inability of the algorithm to converge to a solution. This is due to the fact that depending on the dose distribution resulting from the initialisation, there may not be a compromise solution attainable.

A common approach in RTP is to set the IMB to unity. Such an approach tends to produce an initial distribution that disregards completely the OARs. However, although it has been found that this approach may become trapped in a local optima, it is far superior to a random initialisation for the particular optimisation of IMBs. Note, however, that the approach developed in Chap. 5 to optimise the beam orientation and the beam weight and wedge angle initialises the variable to be optimised randomly to avoid premature convergence [10].

It has been found that the most appropriate initialisation scheme makes use of the dose prescription to determine the first estimate for the IMBs. Indeed this scheme is able to produce consistently good solutions disregarding of the geometry of ROIs, leading to an initial distribution which immediately respects the PTA and OARs.

In order to illustrate this findings, the initial dose distribution obtained by deducing the initial IMBs from the dose prescription for Plan 4.1, is shown in Fig. 4.33. It can be observed that the 90% and 95% isodose lines conform almost exactly to the PTA. However a high dose (above 105%) is observed on the legs of the 'H' shape and a low dose on the edge of the PTA. Figure 4.34 shows the dose distribution obtained after a further 100 iterations of ILS with adaptive weightings. It can be observed that the high dose region has disappeared and that a dose 20% lower than the initial dose is delivered to the OARs.

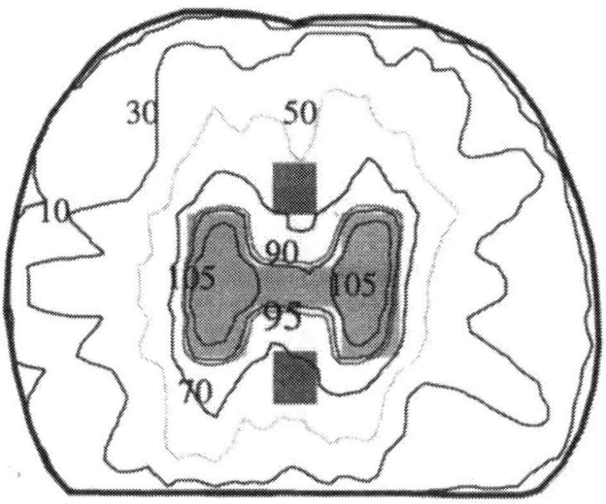

Fig. 4.33 Illustrating the initial dose distribution obtained from the dose prescription by solving the inverse problem

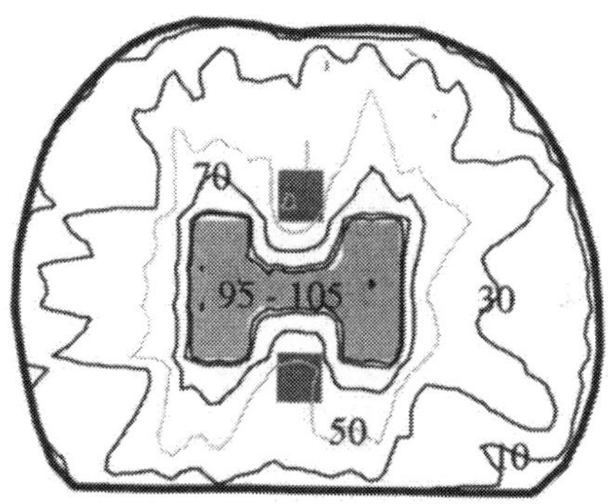

Fig. 4.34 Illustrating the dose distribution obtained after 100 iterations of the ILS scheme with fixed objective weightings

4.6.2 Compensating for Inhomogeneities

As opposed to several other beam models used to optimise IMBs, the beam model developed in this work can account for the presence of inhomogeneities. The aims of this section is first to show that inhomogeneities can be easily accounted for in the solution of the inverse problem and second that they have a significant impact on the resulting IMB profiles. In order to do so a realistic test case, namely Plan 4.2 is used. Recalling Fig. 4.22, the major inhomogeneities in the pelvic regions are the bones on each side of the prostate. These bones are represented by the darkest grey regions in Fig. 4.35.

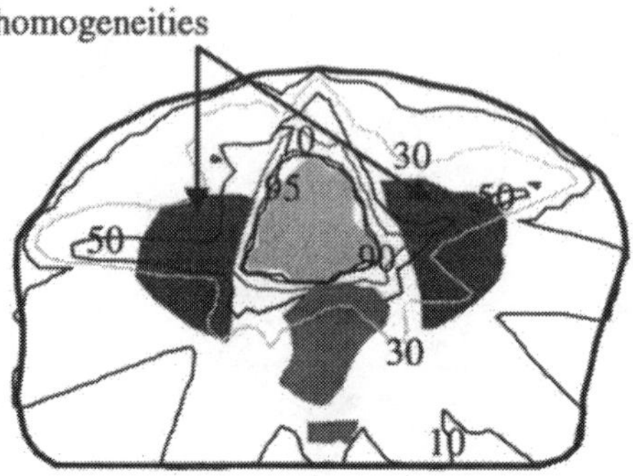

Fig. 4.35 Dose distribution dose (obtained after 100 iterations) for the convex PTA from a prostate plan where the inhomogeneities are not taken into account

Bony structures are characterised by higher densities than the surrounding soft tissues, which results in an increased attenuation of the radiation (see Chap. 2 and 3). In order to demonstrate the principle, the linear attenuation for the bones has been taken as 0.08 cm^{-1}, with the linear attenuation for the other tissues taken as 0.056 cm^{-1} for a 25 MV beam. Dose distributions observed in Fig. 4.35 and 4.36 are similarly acceptable, with a high degree of conformation achieved in the PTA and a very low dose delivered to the OARs.

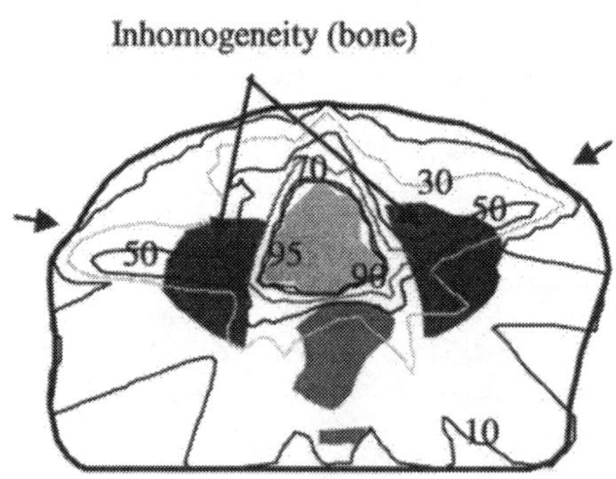

Fig. 4.36 Dose distribution dose (obtained after 100 iterations) for the convex PTA from a prostate plan where the inhomogeneities are taken into account

The main difference between the two plans is that the beams indicated by arrows on Fig. 4.36, which have inhomogeneous regions in their paths, are stronger when inhomogeneities are taken into account. Although the dose incoming from these beams is higher than when inhomogeneities are not taken into account, the isodose contour plots remains very similar around the PTA, thus indicating that the beams have been attenuated in the inhomogeneous regions. This confirms that the beam model designed to solve the inverse problem is able to produce a conformal plan in the presence of inhomogeneities.

This observation is confirmed by Fig. 4.37, where it can be observed that beams 2, 3 and 4 are very similar, but where beams 1 and 5 have higher normalised intensities.

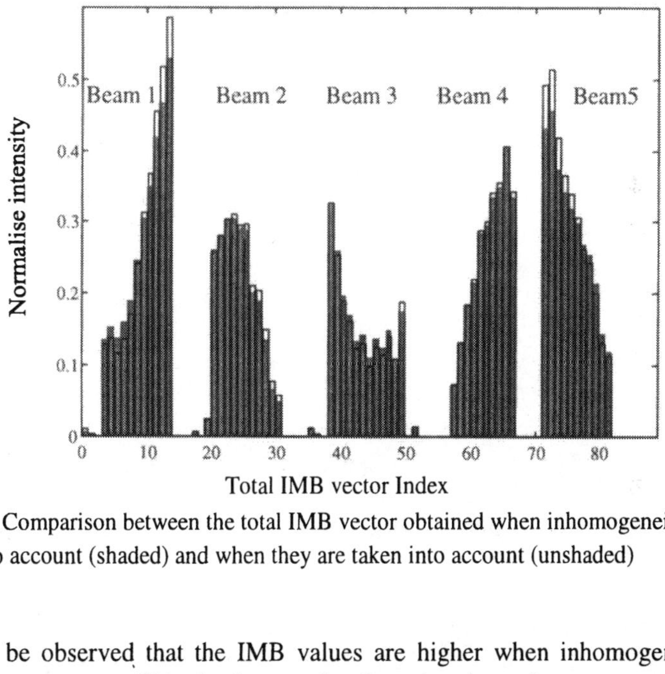

Fig. 4.37 Comparison between the total IMB vector obtained when inhomogeneities are not taken into account (shaded) and when they are taken into account (unshaded)

It can be observed that the IMB values are higher when inhomogeneities are taken into account. This is due to the fact that in order to compensate for inhomogeneities of higher densities, located between the beam entry point and the PTA, it is necessary to increase the intensities of the modulated beams. As such the increased attenuation of the beam is compensated for so that the dose reaching the PTA is as specified.

4.7 Concluding Remarks

Exploiting the matrix formulation of the beam model, Chap. 4 has shown that ILS can perform satisfactorily for both demanding conformal test cases as well as on an actual treatment plan for a patient referred to Walsgrave Hospital. The inclusion of a scalar to modify the elements of the information matrix has shown to improve the performance of the algorithm both in terms of speed of convergence and error. An analogy with the use of forgetting factors and Kalman filtering techniques has been drawn. Provided that the choice of the initial objective weighting factors is appropriate, the weighted sum approach has been shown to perform well, being able to produce high and uniform dose in the PTA whilst delivering a low dose to the OARs. However a poor initial setting of the weighting factors associated with each objective may lead to solutions that are not clinically acceptable or to solutions where *a priori* combination of the objectives is not achievable. Introducing an element of adaptation to evolve the initial choice of objective weightings leads to acceptable solutions, as opposed to optimal solutions, in that the constraints are relaxed or weights reduced when the dose at some particular grid points are considered to be acceptable. This results in adjustment of the trade-off surface, such that the optimisation algorithm attempts to produce a plan where all the criteria are satisfied. This is achieved by concentrating attention towards regions where these criteria are not satisfied whilst disregarding regions where criteria are already satisfied.

It has been highlighted that the solutions produced by the original ILS routine do not ensure that a practicable solution has been determined. In particular depending on the device used to deliver the IMBs, more or less severe constraints may have to be applied.

The inclusion of inhomogeneities in the matrix beam model enables the optimisation of a plan, taking into account inhomogeneous media without any added difficulty. The approach developed in this Chapter, similar to [101], has been demonstrated with parallel beams only. In order to take into account the beam divergence it is required to make use of a variation of the beam model (see Chap. 2 and 3). The extension of the approach to the divergent beam is developed in Chap. 5 and 6.

In this Chap. intensity modulation has been favourably compared to traditional treatment planning techniques. In particular IMBs are able to produce dose distributions that conform more accurately to the PTA whilst ensuring that the OARs do not receive exceedingly high doses. However, in some cases, especially for convex PTA traditional beam shaping techniques may be equally suited to produce acceptable plans provided that a suitable beam orientation is selected.

It may be concluded that the benefits of conformal radiotherapy are not so much in ensuring that the PTA receives the prescribed dose, this can already be achieved by conventional techniques, but also that the OARs and OHT do not receive unacceptably high doses. It is important to re-emphasise that quality of life does not depend so much on the eradication of the cancer at all cost. Indeed harming critical organs may severely impair the quality of life of the patients by causing undesirable side effects [3, 79, 119].

CHAPTER 5
HYBRID GENETIC ALGORITHMS APPLIED TO RADIOTHERAPY TREATMENT PLANNING

5.1 Introduction

In Chap. 4 consideration was given to calculus based optimisation techniques. These techniques have been shown to be useful to solve the inverse problem. However calculus based methods have several drawbacks including the possibility of becoming trapped in local optima and the limitation to objectives formulated in a quadratic form which, given the multi-objective nature of the problem, may not be the optimal formulation.

In the first part of Chap. 5 attention is focused on a heuristic techniques such as genetic algorithms (GAs) which lend themselves well to the optimisation of a number of problems arising in radiotherapy, such as the orientation of the beams, the optimisation of the wedge angles and their corresponding beam weights where the number of variables is relatively small. One of the appealing characteristics of GAs is their robustness and problem independence. In order to improve the performances of a traditional GA, it is possible to adapt several of their attributes to the problem considered by making use of knowledge gained from experience in order to design problem specific operators. Such a process, known as hybridisation, can potentially improve the performances of the GAs for optimising beam weights/wedge angles and coplanar beam orientation in RTP. These two optimisation problems in the field of RTP are likely to have many different objectives to simultaneously satisfy, some of which may be conflicting in nature. This inherent characteristic, which is common to many optimisation problems in RTP has, so far, not been exploited by the search methodologies used to solve these problems. This Chapter presents a novel approach in the field of RTP optimisation; namely that of making use of a multi-objective genetic algorithm (MOGA). Essentially, a MOGA exploits the desirable features of GAs that are suited to solve multi-objective optimisation problems (MOP) [10, 11, 29, 104, 106, 131], with the various objectives being solved in a pseudo parallel fashion during the search. The outcome of the search is then a set of solutions, known as the Pareto optimal set, as opposed to a single solution. A solution, which achieves the best compromise, is then required to be selected from this Pareto optimal set with a decision maker (DM). The advantage of this approach is that it is possible to change the preferences of the DM and select a new optimal solution without having to restart the algorithm.

5.1.1 Guided Random Search

The last fifty years or so, with a particular high growth rate over the last ten years, has seen the rapid development of heuristic and random search strategies which are not based on calculus optimisation methods [132]. This is mainly due to the development of suitable computing facilities together with their abilities to solve non differentiable objective functions. The latter is made possible by the fact that enumerative and guided random search strategies do not require any information about the optimisation problem modelled. These algorithms, that are in a sense problem independent, have been termed '*black box*' algorithms [10, 133]. As such these techniques have been applied to problems which are difficult to model precisely and/or where approximate linear model structures do not hold, i.e. problems with non linear objectives such as the RTP optimisation problem with radiobiological objective functions [30, 89, 120]. These algorithms, which involve an element of randomness, require in general more iterations than calculus based methods; but with the advantage being that each iteration is less computationally demanding, as complex problem specific mathematical models are not required to be developed.

Random based search methods can be divided into two main categories: enumerative and guided random. Enumerative techniques, such as dynamic programming, search the solution space exhaustively evaluating the objective at each point and then deducing directly the optimum [10, 133, 134]. Exhaustive search, which is also referred to as *brute force,* is limited in its application to problems involving a relatively small search space [11, 133].

Guided random search methods can be considered as a major refinement of enumerative techniques. The latter are based on heuristic methods more human like in the sense that they are based on creativity, insight, intuition and learning [1, 133]. These techniques take their inspiration from natural processes and attempt to find the most appropriate combination between exploration (random search, enumerative search) and exploitation (neighbourhood search), where information collected during the search is used to guide the search towards promising regions of the search space (learning) [134]. There are two major types of these heuristic procedures: simulated annealing (SA) and evolutionary algorithms (EA) [10, 131].

SA was first introduced by Metropolis in 1953 [135], and refined by Kirpatrick in 1984 [136]. It is inspired from the annealing process used to bring a substance to its basic state. The process involves heating the substance to melting point and then lowering its temperature slowly enough not to break the system quasi equilibrium [137]. SA performs the exploration by accepting, with a small probability, solutions that may not improve the value of the objective, but which may help escaping a local optima. As the number of iteration increases the search is focused towards a particular region of the search space by progressively reducing the probability of accepting worse solutions. Fast SA (FSA) is similar to SA, but makes use of a Cauchy distribution instead of a Gaussian distribution to generate new solutions. It has been shown to be up to ten times faster than SA for the optimisation of beam weight in RTP [36, 37].

EAs are computer based search techniques inspired from the principle of natural evolution in particular the mechanism of natural selection. EAs as opposed to SA, which uses a single alternative solution at a time, evolve a population of individuals (or alternative solutions) through generations (or iterations) via processes of selection, mutation and reproduction. The major varieties of EAs are: GAs, evolutionary programming (EP), evolution strategies (ES), classifier systems (CS) and genetic programming (GP) [10, 131]. In this work consideration is given to the subset of GAs only.

In RTP, both analytical and random based search techniques have been used [3]. It has been found that analytical search techniques were more efficient to solve the inverse problem where a large number of variables are involved. However, random based search techniques have been shown to perform well in the optimisation of treatment procedures involving the more traditional techniques, such as wedges [4, 30, 37, 87, 88, 89, 90, 92, 120].

5.2 Genetic Algorithms

Originally, GAs were developed at the University of Michigan in the United States and first published by John Holland and his student DeJong in 1975. The aim of their research was to explain adaptive processes of natural systems and design artificial software systems that encompass the important mechanism of natural systems [10, 131]. Because of its origin, the terminology used by the GA community comes from that used in genetics. In order to understand a general description of GAs, it is necessary to explain some specific vocabulary that is employed in a field for which it was not created. The specific meaning of terms borrowed from genetics is fully described in [1].

5.2.1 Simple GA

The original GAs, also known as the simple GA, is defined by Goldberg as "an example of a search procedure that uses random choice to guide highly exploitative search through a coding of parameter space" [134]. In order to design a robust method that could be applicable to a wide variety of problems, a problem independent solving framework had to be developed. This was achieved by using a coded representation of the problem as opposed to the 'real' problem. Working on a coding problem implies that most of the information regarding a particular problem except for the 'pay off', that gives information on the 'goodness' of the solution, is discarded. In addition the operators that provide the means to evolve, or search for a solution, are also problem independent.

GAs make use of adaptive methods inspired by natural evolution and population genetics to solve various combinatorial, classification or optimisation problems, [10, 131, 134]. GAs evolve a group of individuals (called a population) corresponding to alternative solutions for a particular problem by making use of the principle of natural selection borrowed from the Darwinian theory of evolution such as the 'survival of the fittest' principle. GAs explore the search space by selecting solutions to generate future candidate solutions by making use of a probabilistic process, where good solutions are very likely to be selected, but where poor solutions can still be selected. New solutions can be produced by combining or modifying existing solutions via the so called genetic operators [1, 10, 134].

GAs maintain a population of individuals that can be selectively replaced by individuals from a new generation. The use of a population can be thought of as a search in parallel for a solution by investigating alternative solutions in a population.

The mechanisms involved in a simple GA are:

i) *Generate* an initial population of alternative solutions (chromosomes)
ii) *Evaluate* the objective function for each chromosome and deduce the fitness values
iii) *Select* parents from the population according to their fitness to produce offspring
iv) *Combine* each pair of parents together to produce a pair of offspring
v) *Calculate* the objective function and fitness of the new solutions
vi) *Delete* members of the population to *insert* some (or all) of the new solutions into the population
vii) If the stopping criterion is satisfied (the population has converged, or the best solution is within acceptable limits), then stop and return the chromosome with the best ever fitness; otherwise go back to step iii)

The most common methods involved in the population initialisation, the fitness calculation, the recombination and mutation operation and finally the replacement methods are detailed in [1, 10, 131].

5.2.2 Hybridising GAs

Hybridisation is aimed at exploiting the information available in the optimisation procedure to improve the performances of the GAs [131]. The disadvantage is that the introduction of problem specific knowledge specialises the hybrid GA so that it loses some of its problem independent solving characteristics. These adaptations include the use of problem specific coding, such as real values instead of binary, and specialised operators designed to solve a particular problem. The effect of hybridising can be visualised as an attempt to specialise the broad class problem solver, that is to adapt it to a particular niche problem area (see Fig. 5.1). The introduction of problem specific operators to solve for the beam weight/wedge angle and the beam orientation makes the GA less able to solve other problems but provides the user with a more powerful and more appropriate search algorithm.

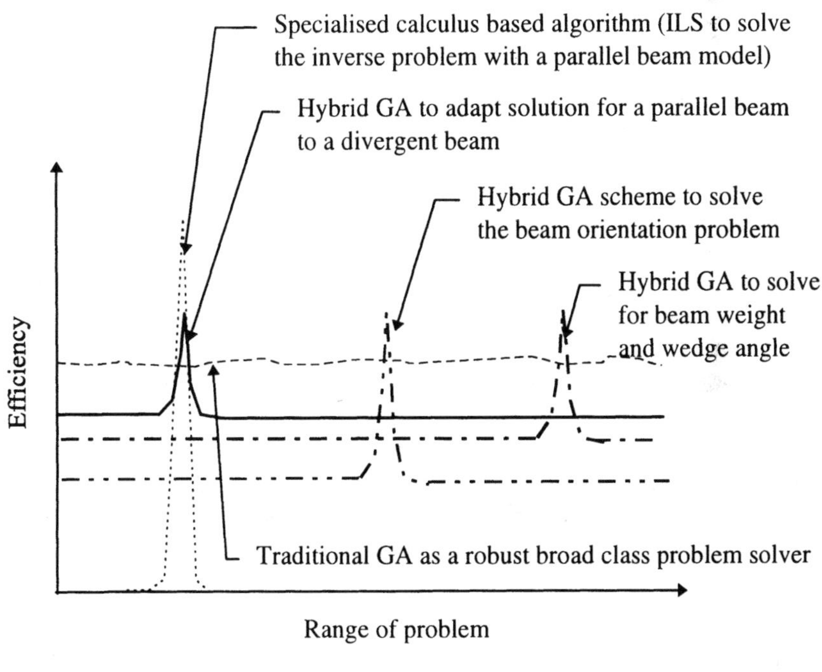

Fig. 5.1 Illustrating the specialisation of hybrid GAs compared to traditional GAs

5.2.3 A Multi-Objective Approach

It has previously been seen that optimisation problems in RTP are very likely to have many objectives, some of which can be conflicting in nature [28]. Various approaches exist to solve for MOPs. According to [138] there are three broad classifications of multi-objective optimisation methods.

The first, which has been used with the ILS scheme, referred to as *a-priori* articulation, makes use of *a-priori* information to combine the different objectives into trade-off functions, that transforms all the objectives into some common measure. In RTP it can be expressed to give a measure of the patient cure, the patient quality of life or a more traditional trade-off function given in terms of dose requirements. However, it has been argued [11, 28, 139] that *a-priori* articulation is equivalent to simplifying the problem into a single objective optimisation problem. Nevertheless this method is the most computationally efficient as all the effort is focused on obtaining a single final trade-off solution right from the beginning of the search. Unfortunately, however, if the final solution, that may be mathematically optimal, is not clinically acceptable, a new combination of the objectives has to be proposed until the optimisation algorithm reaches a clinically acceptable solution. Similarly, if the preference of the DM changes, the algorithm has to be restarted.

The second class, known as *a-posteriori* articulation, determines the set of non dominated solutions, referred to in this work as Pareto optimal set [11, 85, 138], prior to attempting to identify the best compromise solution from that set. The concept of Pareto optimality enables a trade-off solution surface to be found between the various and possibly conflicting objectives. It provides useful information regarding the behaviour of the objectives in relation with each other. In particular it enables the degree to which the objectives are correlated to be determined. If two objectives are correlated, any attempts to solve one objective will also solve the other. In effect it is then possible to reduce the number of objectives to include only those objectives that are in conflict, or orthogonal to each other. Such a thorough investigation of the solution space is made at a higher computational cost. In particular it is necessary to explore all of the solution space in order to determine all non dominated solutions that form the Pareto optimal set, part of which may never be used. This has been reported as a well suited method for static optimisation [1] i.e. where the objectives do not change with time, but where the requirements of the DM may change. In RTP, with each patient being unique, the objectives of the treatment are likely to change with time (here patient by patient, and this may explain why this technique has never been used in RTP).

Remark: It is believed that for certain types of cancer, exhibiting common characteristics, located in a region where the geometry from patient to patient is similar, this method could be used. In fact Pareto optimal sets for typical treatment plans could be used as a starting point of the optimisation for each new patient, which would in effect suppress the need for the search algorithm to perform a lengthy exploration of the solution space before focusing the search.

The third class of multi-objective methods, known as progressive articulation, can be considered as a combination of the previous two, where a DM interacts more closely with the optimisation algorithm, providing a measure of goodness of the proposed solution so that the optimisation algorithm can be used to generate better solutions. It is a compromise between a too narrow and too broad a search.

Compared with the previous approach, the computational cost is lessened at the expense of an increase in complexity of the algorithm, together with an increase in the time required to assess each alternative solution. This approach has previously only received a very limited attention in RTP [89, 119].

Construction of a Decision Maker to Select an Optimal Solution. The type of articulation used in a MOP depends on the problem to be solved, however, common to all these approaches is the need to determine a solution that is optimal for the particular problem to be solved. Indeed, the determination of the trade off surface between all the objectives is only one of the aspect of multi-objective optimisation. The second aspect is the choice of a suitable solution. The most common approaches use:

- weighting coefficients to weight the relative importance of the objectives
- priorities to order the objectives according to their relative importance
- goals to indicate the degree to which the goals are attained

The first approach has been used in Chap. 4 with objectives expressed in a quadratic form such that the inverse problem could be solved with ILS. The use of weighting coefficients is the most common approach to MOP in RTP. The use of weighting coefficients may be considered as the best method, provided that the ideal trade-off is known, however, the last two approaches and in particular the use of priorities may be beneficial in the selection of a solution from a Pareto optimal set (see Sect. 5.3 and 5.4).

5.3 Multi-Objective Genetic Algorithms

A family of EAs aimed at solving MOPs and making use of *a posteriori* or *progressive* articulation is termed a multi-objective genetic algorithm (MOGA). MOGAs are GAs modified to search for solutions of a MOP in parallel by exploiting non dominated solutions exhibiting similar characteristics. There are various methods to handle multiple objectives with GAs, a good review of which can be found in [11]. The approach developed in this work is a Pareto-based approach, similar to that of Fonseca [11, 142], namely Pareto-ranking.

5.3.1 Pareto Ranking

Pareto ranking is a method which makes use of the concept of 'dominance' to differentiate solutions according to the value or cost associated with each of their objectives. Pareto ranking aims to identify all the non dominated solutions which are all optimal, see Fig. 5.2. A solution is said to be non dominated if no improvement can be achieved in the costs associated with any one of the objectives considered. In this work all the non dominated solutions are assigned an identical rank of 1. The rank of the dominated solutions is calculated as follows

$$r = 1 + N_{dominated} \tag{5.1}$$

where r is the rank, $N_{dominated}$ is the number of solutions by which the solution considered is dominated, i.e. the number of solutions which are better than the solution considered for at least one of the objective considered.

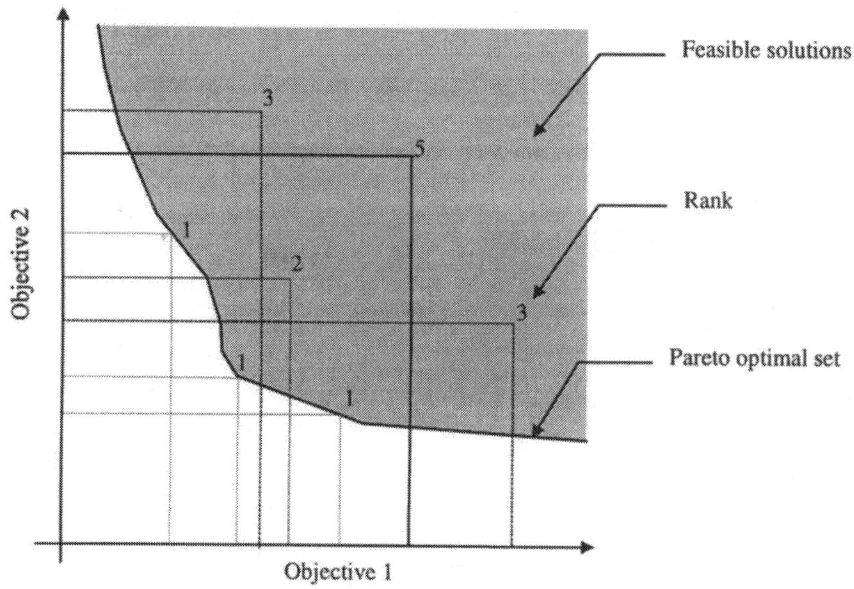

Fig. 5.2 Illustrating Pareto-ranking approach for two objectives

A consequence of the definition of rank adopted in this work is that all the solutions which are dominated by the same number of solutions (or all the non dominated solutions) are associated with an identical rank. For example, it can be observed in the illustrative example of Fig. 5.2, that there are two solutions of rank 3 that are dominated by two solutions that have a smaller cost for both objective 1 and objective 2. A solution of rank 5 is also present that is dominated by four solutions, three of which happen to be of rank one and one of rank two. However, there is no solution of rank 4 because none of the solutions represented is dominated by three other solutions. This redundancy or absence of a particular rank is one of the main difference between Pareto ranking and traditional ranking methods.

5.3.2 Selection Methods

The simplest method to select individuals from the current population is to use traditional rank based fitness assignment methods, with the sole difference being that the rank is not related to the position of an individual with respect to its objective but is now given by equation (5.1). Such an approach could lead, after a few generations, to a population composed solely of non dominated solutions and therefore to individuals having the same rank of unity, leading to an identical probability of being selected. At this stage, the selection of a new individual would become a random process. However, in most problems, solutions located at one extreme of the Pareto set may be very different to solutions located at the other. It is generally accepted that a combination of these two solutions is not likely to give rise to a better individual [11, 28, 131, 139]. Therefore it is necessary to differentiate individuals of similar rank, such that the combination of individuals that are more likely to produce improved solutions is favoured. This can be achieved, to some extent, by the so called 'niching' methods [131, 139].

Progressive Articulation with Pareto Ranking. In this work the aim is to focus the search on region(s) of the search space that is/are likely to offer an acceptable solutions. However the shape of the solution space and, therefore, the trade-off that can be achieved is not common to all treatment plans in RTP. Consequently it may not be easy to identify the 'best', in some sense, region of the Pareto optimal set that is likely to offer the most favourable compromise. Therefore a scheme that enables sufficient degree of freedom to either investigate all the Pareto optimal set (when no a priori information is available) or to concentrate on a particular region of this set has been adopted. It makes use of a DM to differentiate solutions with identical rank.

By keeping the preferences of the DM fixed, the search concentrates on the region indicated by the DM, whilst being able to produce non-dominated solutions in other regions of the search space; thus keeping a small level of exploration together with the exploitation of a particular region. Indeed the selection being a heuristic process, although solutions favoured by the DM may have a higher chance of being selected, other non-dominated solutions can still be selected with a small probability.

The DM may also change its preferences as the search progresses in a deterministic or a heuristic manner. This enables the focus of the search on different regions of the solution space to change, therefore enabling a better exploration of the search space than the previous approach. In this work the following approaches to articulate/combine the objectives have been investigated:

- Alternating the objectives randomly
- At each iteration only one objective is considered by setting its objective weighting to unity, the other objective weightings being set to zero. The particular objective considered at each iteration is chosen randomly.
- Alternating the objectives sequentially in an orderly manner

- Similar to the previous method, but where the objectives are chosen in a sequential manner.
- Random combination of the objectives
- Each objective weighting is chosen randomly, such that the DM is a weighted sum of the objectives that evolves in a random manner. By making use of additional scalar weightings, it is possible to emphasise the relative importance of some objectives.

These techniques which have been used to direct the search as it progresses can also be used at a later stage to select the optimal solution from the Pareto optimal set. However, in many cases goals have been used to select the appropriate solution from the Pareto optimal set. The approach usually involves the setting of a minimal requirement for the cost in the PTA and then the selection of the optimal solution according to the cost in the OAR, with variation of the cost in the OHT being used to differentiate between similar solutions.

The DM used in conjunction with the MOGA to guide the search combines the normalised cost of the various objectives, such that the fitness:

$$\text{Fitness} = r + \alpha f_{DM}(O_1, O_2, \ldots O_n) \tag{5.2}$$

where the scalar quantity $0 < \alpha < 1$ is chosen to emphasise the relative importance of the rank and the output of the decision maker f_{DM} which is of the form:

$$f_{DM}(O_1, O_2, \ldots O_n) = \sum_{i=1}^{n}\left(\lambda_i \frac{O_i}{M_i}\right) \Bigg/ \sum_{i=1}^{n}(\lambda_i) \tag{5.3}$$

where n, $\lambda_i \in \Re^+$, O_i and $M_i > 0$, $i = 1 \ldots n$, are, respectively, the number of objectives, the objective weightings, the values of each objective and the maximum value of a given objective in the current population.

Remark: An interesting feature of MOGA is that objectives of a different nature that are difficult to combine into a single cost function can still be solved simultaneously. It could be particularly interesting to combine, therefore, physical objectives based on dose requirements with other objectives based on radiobiological considerations such as tumour control probability (TCP) and normal tissue control probability (NTCP), as well as that of the patient quality of life. Such an approach may assist in the design of an optimal objective function that can give a more accurate prediction on the actual quality of the treatment planned.

5.3.3 Diagramatic Representation

The overall optimisation approach making use of the MOGA with progressive articulation of the objective and a posteriori selection of the most suitable solution is summarised in Fig. 5.3.

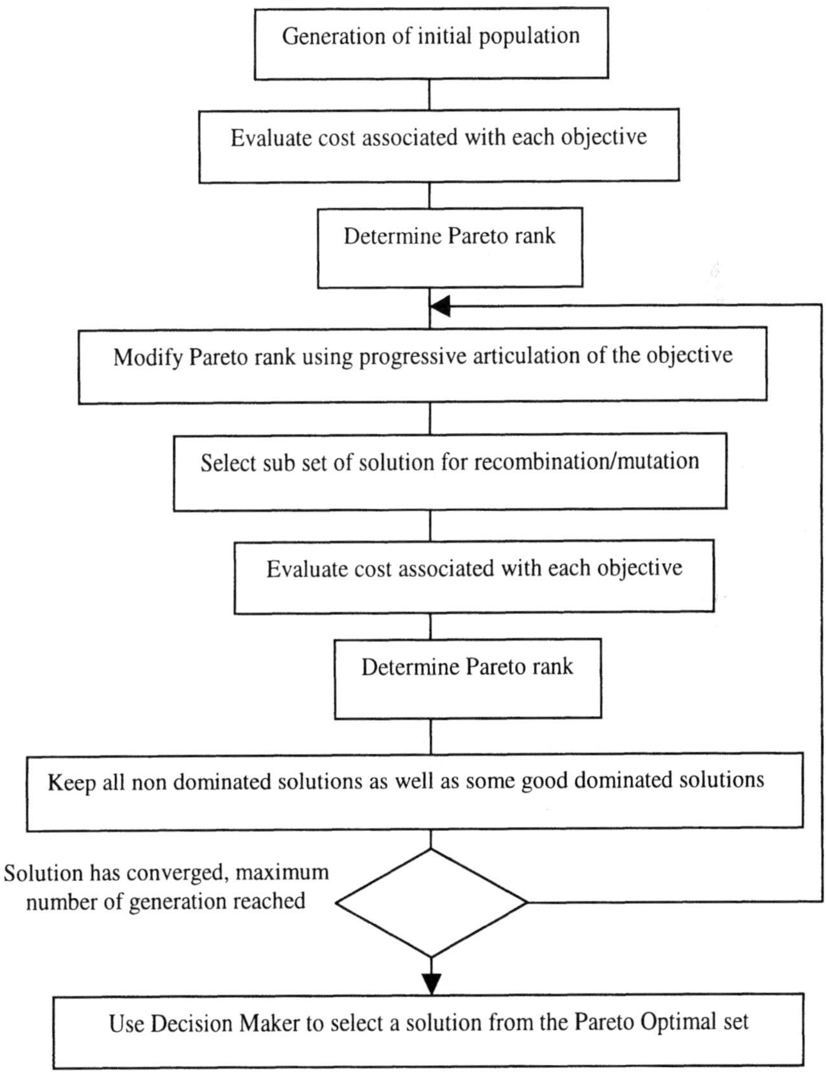

Fig. 5.3 Illustrating the MOGA approach with Pareto Ranking and progressive articulation of the objective

5.4 Optimisation of Coplanar Beam Orientation in Radiotherapy

This section describes the use of a hybridised version of the MOGA introduced in Sect. 5.3 to solve for the coplanar beam orientation in RTP. The solution of the beam orientation problem involves the determination of the gantry angle and, therefore, the beam entry point for each beam used in the treatment. The optimal solution depends on several clinical factors such as the accessibility of the PTA, the respective location of the PTA and the OARs, the avoidance of critical organs and more generally the patient geometry together with some empirical knowledge regarding the benefits or the effectiveness of particular beam settings such as for example the hinged pair and the three field brick. This problem attempts to solve simultaneously several competing objectives and is treated as a MOP. A novel geometrical objective function is formulated which attempts to replicate the approach of a treatment planner. It involves the mapping of the traditional objectives based on dose requirements onto geometrical objectives based on the area of the ROIs covered by individual beams. When the approach is applied without constraining the number of beams, the solution to the beam orientation problem also produces, as a by-product; namely an indication of the minimum number of beams required. Alternatively the Pareto optimal approach that is used to solve this MOP offers the possibility to determine the Pareto optimal set for various number of beams simultaneously.

Hybrid operators are introduced with the aim of 'speeding up' the MOGA by exploiting empirical knowledge in order to reduce the number of times the objective functions are required to be calculated whilst, at the same time, improve the accuracy of the solution. Integer coded GAs are used together with traditional and application specific operators.

The geometrical approach is first assessed on standard test cases prior to its demonstration on an actual medical problem. It is shown that the novel geometrical formulation leads to optimised plans, giving rise to improved dose distributions.

5.4.1 Brief Review of Existing Approaches - Orientation

The coplanar beam orientation problem has been solved with various methods, see for example [3, 27, 29, 30, 80]. Some are calculus based, others make use of guided random search techniques or the rather more enumerative techniques.

Godkhale *et al* [29] has used an analytical technique similar to that used to solve the inverse RTP problem to optimise beam orientation in rotation therapy. This approach is based on determining the 'path of least resistance' from a fictitious radiation source located at the centre of the tumour. The radiation source is assumed to emit radiation in all directions. Adopting such an approach, the point with the highest dose on the surface corresponds to the position which has been reached by the photon emitted with less effort following the path of least resistance. The optimised beam gantry angles correspond to the angles made by lines joining the points with the highest dose on the surface to the fictitious source of the radiation. The advantage of this method is that, as opposed to the other iterative methods [3, 27] it only requires one step to determine the dose at the patient surface. The disadvantage is that it may favour parallel opposed beams for almost symmetrical targets, which have been shown by other workers [3] not to be the optimal beam configuration in conformation therapy, where complex beam modulation and shaping devices are available.

More standard optimisation techniques have also been used in conjunction with radiobiological objectives [3, 30, 80, 140, 141] and objectives based on dose criteria [1, 27, 30]. In both cases, it was observed that the solution space for the beam orientation problem was composed of a large number of local optima. Söderström *et al* [80, 141] demonstrated the latter with radiobiological objective function by performing a semi exhaustive search on two beams of a three beam plan; with a beam already fixed in its optimal position at $\theta = 0°$, where θ is the beam gantry angle, and the remaining two allowed to vary in 10° intervals. The presence of so many local optima has rightly prompted Söderström *et al* into deducing that: "for this type of optimisation problem, a gradient algorithm may be inadequate since it could get trapped in some of the many local maxima" [3, 80]. The optimisation of only two gantry angles (one beam fixed) with a precision limited to a 10° interval required 20 days calculation time on a HP 9000 and this to evaluate only 666 different combinations, where, each new beam configuration required 45 min to be evaluated. This is due to the fact for each new beam orientation, optimal beam profiles had to be calculated with a full beam model including scatter and inhomogeneities [80, 141].

In order to reduce the time required to evaluate the objective function at each iteration, Bortfled *et al* [27] have used a simplified parallel beam model, where only the primary contribution is modelled using an exponential function, therefore, disregarding the effect of scatter. The approach followed by Bortfled *et al* combines FSA with an objective function based on dose criteria. In order to further reduce the time required to evaluate the objective function, the latter is represented in the frequency domain. However, such an approach is limited to a least square objective function where the sum of the squares of the error between the prescribed and the calculated dose is minimised.

Other studies determine sub optimal beam orientation by starting the optimisation of beam profiles with a relatively large number of equispaced beams (36 in Morill *et al* [88]) and progressively reducing the number of beams involved in the plan by removing beams accounting for only a small contribution to the overall dose delivered to the patient. The latter approaches do not directly optimise the beam orientation but rather eliminate non optimal beam orientations to reduce the number of beams to a practicable number. The problem with such approaches is that the relatively small number of gantry angles originally present does not allow the optimisation algorithms to explore the entire search space.

5.4.2 Motivation for the Geometrical Approach

The lessons that can be learned from the previous approaches are as follows. The solution space of the coplanar beam orientation problem is composed of a large number of local optima, which imply that gradient descent methods are not well suited to solve such a problem. Therefore alternative optimisation techniques such as those inspired from SA or EAs are required.

It has been observed that making use of such heuristic techniques may require many thousands of function evaluations [104]. In order to reduce the time required to determine an acceptable solution it is possible to:

- reduce the time required to evaluate the objective function (e.g. use of simplified beam models)
- reduce the number of iterations necessary to obtain an acceptable solution.

The latter may imply the use of some *a priori* knowledge in the optimisation algorithm. For this reason the use of EAs such as GAs is favoured. As opposed to SA, a GA makes use of genetic search operators that can be hybridised to include problem specific information, thus potentially improving the search process whilst maintaining the overall advantages of the evolutionary approach. To further speed up the process in this work, a novel geometrical formulation of the objective has been proposed [28, 139].

Although some of the methods developed to automatically optimise the beam orientation problem have been shown to perform satisfactorily, the treatment planners and clinicians are still today applying manual techniques in the positioning of beams. This is due to the fact that in most cases human operators can very easily predict and visualise the geometrical arrangement of a few coplanar beams. However, it is much easier for a computer to determine accurately the overall dose distribution resulting from a given manual beam setting than it is for a human. One of the reasons for the human to perform so fast is that in most cases it is not necessary to calculate the total distribution to assess a possible beam setting; with use being made of the RTP software mainly to verify a particular beam configuration. From time to time the treatment planner will be required to modify the beam orientation after his/her initial estimation but only by a small amount. However, when the number of beams increases, the treatment planner encounters difficulties in producing an optimal plan, although it is possible to produce sub-optimal but acceptable plans after a few trials.

The approach proposed in this work attempts to replicate the procedure followed by the treatment planners by making use of objectives based on geometrical considerations. The approach differs from [3, 27, 30, 80, 140, 141] in that it does not require the calculation of the total dose distribution for each new beam gantry angle nor the solution of the inverse problem for each new beam setting (see Chap. 4). However, in some cases, in order to determine the optimal solution for a particular patient, it may be required to evaluate the total dose distribution for solutions lying on the Pareto optimal set and solve the inverse problem or optimise the wedge angles/beam weights. This lengthy process is only involved at a later stage in the optimisation procedure, and the determination of the Pareto optimal set only involves the use of geometrical relationships and planar image processing techniques to determine areas created by the intersection of the beam paths with the ROI. This geometrical approach results in a reduction in the amount of operations that are required to evaluate the objectives at each function call.

In order to be able to predict accurately and clinically optimal beam settings, geometrical objectives have to relate to more traditional objectives based on dose requirements. In this work four objectives are considered. The first three are related to the traditional objectives of RTP, i.e. delivering a high and uniform dose in the PTA, a low dose in the OHT and in particular in the OARs. A further objective is the number of beams.

The traditional approach is to make use of some *a priori* knowledge to design a utility function that offers the best compromise. However, in this case the nature of the objectives is quite different which complicates such design.

As opposed to all the previous approaches that offer only a single solution to the optimisation of beam orientation, the approach adopted in this work enables the clinician to choose between several alternative solutions involving a variable number of beams. This is believed to offer an additional advantage in that, in some cases, a different number of beams than the number originally specified by the clinicians may be more appropriate.

Although the approach developed in this work is valid for coplanar beams only, a similar approach could also be used with non coplanar beams, by replacing the planar geometry used by space geometry and volumetric information. The latter, however, would result in an execution time of the algorithm being significantly larger due to the increased computational burden and increased dimensionality of the solution space. Indeed this is a clear area for immediate further work.

5.4.3 Geometrical Formulation: Preliminaries

In order to simplify and automate the calculation of various areas involved in the evaluation of the objectives, ROIs and beam paths are represented by polygons. Four types of polygons are used. The simplest polygon, represented by four pairs of point co-ordinates, outlines the area covered by a beam path. This enables, without increasing the mathematical complexity of the objective function, the consideration of either parallel or divergent beams [28, 126, 139] (see Fig. 5.4). A beam is represented by a polygon as follows:

$$B = \begin{bmatrix} x_1 & x_2 & x_3 & x_4 \\ y_1 & y_2 & y_3 & y_4 \end{bmatrix} \tag{5.4}$$

where B is the polygon describing the beam path as a trapezium defined by four points B_1, B_2, B_3 and B_4 (see Fig. 5.4) which co-ordinates are given respectively by (x_1,y_1), (x_2,y_2), (x_3,y_3) and (x_4,y_4). Note that the polygon B contains four pairs of co-ordinates. $FS = [B_1\ B_2]$ is the field size of the beam at the skin level, chosen such that it encompass all the target region in addition to two small margins to account for the beam penumbra. The co-ordinates of the beam polygons are deduced from the position of the isocentre, denoted I, the source to skin distance, denoted SSD and the field size FS of the beam.

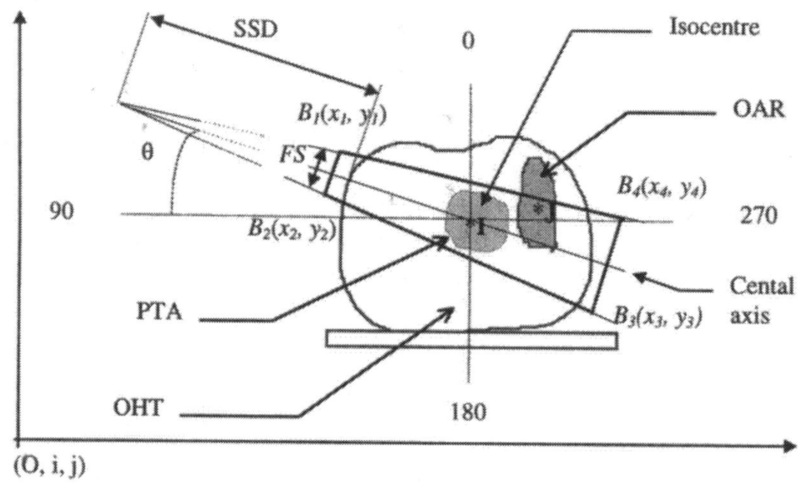

Fig. 5.4 Polygonal representation of a beam in the transaxial (xy) plane with arbitrary location of PTA and OAR for purpose of illustration

Other polygons used to describe the contours of the ROIs and the patient contour contain more points as they describe more complex geometrical shapes. Note that the number of points should be kept to a minimum to speed up the evaluation of the objectives without losing too much accuracy. It can be observed in Fig. 5.4 that the polygons defining the PTA and the OARs are included within the polygon defining the patient contour. For coplanar beam orientation, the planning is usually performed on the most representative slice, and the PTA is determined such that the extent of the disease in all the slices involved in the planning process is encompassed. For 3-D coplanar beam orientation, several parallel slices can be considered, where for each slice new polygons are used to describe the ROIs and the patient body contour.

In this work unless stated otherwise, the planning is assumed to be carried out on a single slice which is considered to be the most representative. It is also assumed that variation of the size of the PTA along the patient head to toe axis is taken care of by beam shaping devices such as multi-leaf collimators (MLCs) [3].

5.4.4 Formulation of the Objectives - Orientation

The usual assessment of a radiotherapy plan is made on criteria involving dose received by different regions within the patient. In the geometrical approach adopted it is necessary to reformulate these objectives in terms of geometrical relationships. This section reviews the theoretical basis for the new geometrical formulation of some RTP objectives involved in the coplanar beam orientation problem.

Conforming to the PTA. In the beam orientation problem it is not necessary to include into the objectives the dose uniformity requirement in the PTA which can be achieved by optimising the beam shapes and profiles. However, the formulation of the objective should reflect the need for the combination of beams to conform to the PTA. Therefore, the first objective calculates the discrepancy between the area where all the beams overlap and the area of the PTA such that the cost relating to the PTA, denoted C_{PTA} is given by:

$$C_{PTA} = (area(B_1 \cap B_2 \cdots \cap B_{N_{Beam}}) - area(\mathrm{PTA}))^k \tag{5.5}$$

where B_i, i=1...N_{Beam} are the polygons representing the individual beam paths and k is an integer, $k \in \aleph^+$, used to emphasise small differences in areas. Note that k is only useful when the various objectives are combined. When the objectives are solved in parallel, k can be kept to unity.

Note that all these areas are calculated by determining the area of polygons resulting from the intersection of the beams. It is also interesting to note that the area covered by the PTA is required to be calculated only once. In addition, the position of the PTA with respect to the beam overlap regions does not have to be recorded as the PTA is always totally included in each beam path and therefore in the area where all the beams overlay.

Minimising High Dose to the OHT. It has been seen previously that the planning should ensure that a low dose is delivered to the OHTs. However, high dose regions may occur for two reasons. First, when use is made of a small number of beams (i.e. two or three), and the PTA is located deep into the body, hot spots may occur near the beam entry point at x_{max}. Provided that no higher beam energy is available, the only plausible solution to this problem is to increase the number of beams, so that the portion allocated to each beam is reduced, thus reducing the risk of creating hot spots. However, increasing the number of beams is also likely to increase the area of tissues affected by radiation. Therefore a compromise has to be reached between irradiating a large area with a low dose or a smaller area with a larger dose. This issue is not directly considered in this work as it depends on several clinical factors. However, the Pareto optimal formulation enables the inclusion of such factors in the selection of the 'best' plan at a later stage.

A high dose can also occur when several beams overlay outside the PTA. In order to overcome this problem, it is possible to modulate the beam intensity. The simplest method is to ensure that the area of overlay is minimised outside the PTA. This can be achieved by minimising the following expression of the cost relating to the OHTs, denoted C_{OHT}, given by:

$$C_{OHT} = \sum_{i=1}^{n-1} \sum_{j=i+1}^{n} area(B_i \cap B_j) \tag{5.6}$$

Which represent the sum of all the areas of beam overlap outside the PTA, between each pair of beams involved in the plan. This is aimed to penalise parallel opposed beams, or beams with similar gantry angles that have an important area of overlap.

Note that this calculation may be a lengthy process as it is necessary to calculate the co-ordinates of the polygons resulting from the beam intersection prior to calculating its area. In order to speed up the calculation of C_{OHT}, parallel beams are assumed. The intersection made by two parallel beams is then a parallelogram and its area is equal to the product of the base by the height. It can be deduced that the area formed by two intersecting beams B_i and B_j is given by:

$$Area(B_i \cap B_j) = \begin{cases} \dfrac{w_i w_j}{\left|\sin(\theta_i - \theta_j)\right|}, \theta_i \neq \theta_j \\ 2 * Area(B_i), \theta_i = \theta_j \end{cases} \tag{5.7}$$

where w_i, θ_i and w_j, θ_j are the width and the angle of beam i and j respectively.

Minimising Exposure of OARs. The aim of this objective is to reduce the dose that can potentially be delivered to the OARs. This may be interpreted as minimising the area of beam overlap with each OAR. Provided that a particular OAR can be totally spared, a null cost could then be achieved. However, depending on the location of the OAR it may be impossible to avoid them. In this case, it may be advantageous to minimise the volume of the region of the OAR receiving radiation, even if the dose received by this small region is relatively high. (This may occur if only a few beams are involved in a plan, or if several beams overlap over the OAR.) Alternatively it may be better to ensure that a larger region of the OAR is irradiated but with a much lower dose. The latter can be achieved by increasing the number of beams involved in a plan and ensuring that only a minimum number of beams deliver a dose to the OAR. From this observation it is concluded that the cost in the OAR should be inversely proportional to the number of beams involved in a plan.

Finally, one of the most efficient methods to reduce the amount of radiation received by an OAR, where use is made of traditional radiotherapy techniques, is to ensure that the beam entry point is as distant from the OAR as is physically possible, thus enabling the dose to be attenuated by the tissues it traverses. However, it has recently been found, see [140, 141], that when use is made of IMRT with plan including a concave PTA enclosing an OAR in the pelvic region, the optimal beam arrangement for a five field plan involved a posterior beam directly facing the spine. Despite the fact that these findings goes against current practices, it is shown in Stein *et al* [141], that it is easier to control the dose in a concave PTA when a beam entry point is closer to the concave region and, therefore, the critical structure within the PTA concavity.

In order to incorporate all these requirements, two different formulation were adopted. The traditional formulation is aimed at radiotherapy techniques making use of simple beam modulation devices such as wedges. The modified formulation is aimed at IMRT, which can modulate the beams to achieve conformal treatments. In both cases, the cost associated with the OAR, denoted C_{OAR}, is given by

$$C_{OAR} = \rho \sum_{i=1}^{n} \frac{area(B_i \cap \mathrm{OAR})}{N_{beam}}, \tag{5.8}$$

For the traditional formulation $\rho \in \Re^+$ is given by

$$\begin{cases} \delta_{OAR} < \delta_{PTA}, \rho = \beta(\delta_{PTA} - \delta_{OAR}) \\ \delta_{OAR} \geq \delta_{PTA}, \rho = 1 \end{cases} \tag{5.9}$$

where δ_{OAR} is the distance between the projection of the centre '*J*' of the OAR onto the CAX and the beam entry point, δ_{PTA} is the distance between the isocentre '*I*' of the PTA and the beam entry point and $\beta \in \Re^+$, β is a user defined parameter chosen such that $\beta(\delta_{PTA}\text{-}\delta_{OAR}) > 1$.

For the modified formulation $\rho = 1$, however, the polygons B_i describing the individual beam path are modified to account for the fact that with IMRT it is possible to block part of the field which are facing OARs. It has been observed that the closer an OAR the greater is the modulation in beam intensity, and the lower is the intensity of the elemental beams facing the OAR considered. In order to reflect this finding, individual beams B_i are split when the distance from the centre of the OAR to the beam entry points is smaller than the distance between the isocentre and the beam entry point. This allow a total sparing of the OAR directly facing the beams.

Note that it is convenient to assume from a geometrical view point that the beams still encompass the PTA, the individual split beams are only used to calculate the cost for the OARs using equation (5.8).

5.4.5 Coding Considerations - Orientation

With binary coding the main problem is that in order to achieve the required accuracy many bits are required and, depending on the range of the variable, part of the chromosome may not contain useful information. For example in the beam orientation problem in RTP, each beam angle θ lies in a range such that $\theta \in [0\ 359°]$. Using a binary system 9 bits representing a variable in the range [0 511°] would be required. Consequently the binary coded variables between 360° and 511° do not correspond to a possible solution. In order to overcome this problem an integer representation is used, thus eliminating the need for coding and decoding each variable. Given the actual degree of accuracy of the beam orientation mechanism, a resolution for θ of 1° (i.e. $\theta \in \aleph$) is considered sufficient for practicable implementation. Making use of an integer representation gives rise to a much shorter chromosome; the length of each chromosome being equal to the number of beams involved in the plan, i.e. a chromosome $C \in \aleph^N$ which corresponds to a particular solution is represented as a vector $C^T = [\ \theta_1, \theta_2, \ldots \theta_N\ ]$, where the θ_i, $i=1, 2, \ldots N$, denote the beam angles.

As an example, consider the arbitrary case of four beams displaced as shown in Table 5.1. This shows the relationship between the physical value and its binary coded representation together with its actual integer value. Note that in the case of integer coding, the physical value of the angle and its coded representation are identical, thus removing the need for coding and decoding. The chromosomes in each case are represented by the concatenation of the coded representation of each beam.

Table 5.1 Relation between coded representation and physical meaning of the variables involved in the optimisation of coplanar beam orientation in RTP

Variable (gantry angle)	Beam 1	Beam 2	Beam 3	Beam 4
Physical value	0°	130°	300°	270°
Binary coding	000000000	010000010	100101100	100001110
Integer coding	0	130	300	270
Chromosome (binary coding)	000000000010000010100101100100001110			
Chromosome (integer coding)	0 130 300 270			

5.4.6 Hybridisation by Inclusion of Problem Specific Search Operators

Intermediate Crossover. A traditional crossover operator that exchanges parts of the parents [1] would not be able to explore new regions of the search space when use is made of integer coding because it cannot produce new integers. One solution adopted to improve the performance of the crossover operator is to modify operators used with real coded GAs [131, 142] such as for example intermediate recombination. Such operators can produce new possible solutions that lie in regions of the solution space slightly larger than that defined by the parents to ensure that the offspring produced are integer valued, such that the new operator follows the rule

$$C_O = \text{round}(C_{P1} + \gamma\,(C_{P2} - C_{P1})) \tag{5.10}$$

where $\gamma \in \Re$ is a random number that lies in the interval [-0.25 1.25] [142], and C_{P1} and C_{P2} denotes the parents selected from the population. The bounds of the intervals have been chosen to provide a good compromise between exploration and exploitation.

Mutation. The mutation operator introduces new beam angles into the search space by generating integers that lie in the range [0 359°] for divergent beams or [0 179°] for parallel beams.

Problem Specific Operators. To exploit the specific features of the beam orientation problem, operators which attempt to replicate the traditional approach followed by human operators have been introduced. The first problem specific operator selects one existing beam orientation randomly or creates a new gantry angle and then positions the remaining beams evenly. This has been designed from the consideration that equispaced beams irradiate a large volume with a low dose whilst giving a high dose to the target. Although equispaced beams may not be the optimal beam configuration, they have been shown to be near-optimal [3, 27, 80, 140, 141]. In addition, when the algorithm is used to minimise the number of beams as well as their orientation, the operator produces equispaced beams for the various combinations of beams in the range: $N_{min} \leq k \leq N_{max}$, where k is the number of beams not replicated within a chromosome with $2 \leq N_{min}$ and $N_{max} \leq N$. This operator makes use of a single parent C_{P1} to produce one offspring C_O with the following rule:

$$C_{P1} = [\theta_1\ \theta_2 \ldots \theta_N]$$

gives $$C_O = \left[\theta_i \quad \left(\theta_i + \frac{2\pi}{k}\right) \quad \cdots \quad \left(\theta_i + \frac{2(k-1)\pi}{k}\right) \quad \theta_a \quad \cdots \quad \theta_a\right] \tag{5.11}$$

with $\theta_i \in \{\theta_1\ \theta_2 \ldots \theta_N\}$ if chosen from an existing chromosome

or $\theta_i \in [0, 359]$ if randomly generated

where θ_a is a gantry angle of superfluous beams, i.e. duplications of gantry angles

and $$\theta_a \in \left\{\theta_i, \quad \left(\theta_i + 2\frac{\pi}{k}\right), \quad \cdots \quad \left(\theta_i + \frac{2(k-1)\pi}{k}\right)\right\}$$

in which the number of beams k lies in the range $2 \leq k \leq 5$, as only minor improvements can be achieved when $k > 5$ [140].

This operator may produce a few identical gantry angles. Although these redundant gantry angles are ignored in the evaluation of a given solution, they may be involved in exchange or modification of the chromosome, such that beams which provide potentially good solutions are spread more rapidly into the rest of the population. Provided that these beams are optimal this is advantageous, however, in cases where they are only sub-optimal it may become a drawback. An alternative method would be to regenerate random beams each time redundant beams are encountered. This would result in a better exploration of the solution space, at the cost of a slower rate of convergence. In RTP with the computing resources being limited, it is found to be more favourable to obtain rapid exploitation of good solutions as opposed to a more thorough exploration.

Note that when the number of beams is not minimised (i.e. $k = N$) an operator ensures that each beam gantry angle within a chromosome is unique, such that $\theta_a \in \{\}$.

The second problem specific operator shifts all the beams by a small amount $\delta\theta$, mainly in order to speed up the final stage of the optimisation to fine tune the beam orientation such that a parent C_{P1} gives rise to a unique offspring C_O such that:

$$C_{P1} = [\theta_1 \; \theta_2 \ldots \theta_N] \text{ becomes } C_O = [(\theta_1 + \delta\theta) \; (\theta_2 + \delta\theta) \ldots (\theta_N + \delta\theta)] \tag{5.13}$$

The third problem specific operator acts similarly to the mutation operator, but is limited to a small range of values. It shifts one beam gantry angle θ_i, i=1...N selected randomly by a small amount (less than 15°) such that:

$$C_{P1} = [\theta_1 \; \theta_2 \ldots \theta_N] \text{ becomes } C_O = [\theta_1 \; \theta_2 \ldots (\theta_i + \delta\theta) \ldots \theta_N] \tag{5.14}$$

It has been observed during the research that the algorithm can find relatively quickly the correct beam path, however, it may encounter some difficulty in determining the optimal beam entry point. In order to overcome this problem, a fourth problem specific operator is introduced. It adds 180° to a beam i, i=1...N chosen randomly such that:

$$C_{P1} = [\theta_1 \; \theta_2 \ldots \theta_N] \text{ becomes } C_O = [\theta_1 \; \theta_2 \ldots (\theta_i + 180) \ldots \theta_N] \tag{5.15}$$

It is only used when divergent beams are considered with an alphabet coding for all the beam orientations between 0° and 359°. Indeed when parallel beams are assumed, the beam angles θ and $\theta + \pi$ are identical and it is only necessary to code angles in the range [0 179°]. The result of the optimisation is then an optimal beam path, but no attempt is made to determine the best beam entry point. The beam entry points could be determined afterwards by the clinicians or by calculating the dose distribution and dose area histogram.

When solving the beam orientation problem the algorithm may converge to a solution where many beams are superimposed, thus leading to a reduced number of independent beam paths. In order to determine the optimum combination of beams, each beam is required to be unique. Therefore once the above operators have been used the angles are constrained to lie in the range [0 179°] (for parallel beams) or [0 359°] (for divergent beams), i.e. an offspring C^T=[100 370 420] in a three beam configuration becomes C^T=[100 10 60].

An advantage of these operators is that they are fast to compute. A disadvantage lies in the fact that at least N_{min} new beam angles in the solution are required to be unique where $N_{min} \leq N$ is the minimum number of beams specified by the clinicians, therefore it is necessary to constrain the beams between the predefined range to ensure that two beams are not physically identical although being numerically different (i.e. 0° = 360°).

5.4.7 Simulation Studies – Beam Orientation

The aim of the simulation studies is to show that the geometrical approach is able to replicate generally accepted beam settings for standard treatment plans as well as beam arrangements use in IMRT. Various test cases introduced in Chap. 4 are also used to demonstrate the ability of the algorithm to determine clinically acceptable solutions. The geometrical approach is then validated by comparing dose distributions resulting from an optimised and a more traditional beam setting, for a typical treatment plan corresponding to an actual patient.

Ability to Reproduce Beam Settings Used for Standard Plans. Conventional treatment of cancer in the pelvic region leads to 'boxed in' square or rectangular shapes, i.e. the PTA is arbitrarily taken as a square or a rectangle. In order to test the proposed orientation algorithm a plan, subsequently referred to as Plan 5.1, involving a square PTA is used. Figure 5.5 shows the optimised beam settings for a three and a four field plan. As expected, the beam arrangement that conforms more accurately to the PTA involves beams positioned at right angles. The three field plan makes use of one posterior beam and two parallel opposed beams, whereas, the four field plan uses two pairs of parallel opposed beams.

It can be observed that the optimised gantry angles are not exactly positioned at 0, 90, 180 and 270 degrees due to the fact that the optimisation algorithm attempts to reproduce the PTA shapes and therefore in order to produce square angles with divergent beams it is necessary to modify the beam orientation slightly so that one edge of the beam is parallel to one edge of the square PTA. Trials on rectangular PTA have also shown that when three beams are used the parallel opposed beams are parallel to the longest side of the PTA which ensures a better match between the PTA and the region of beam overlap (RBO).

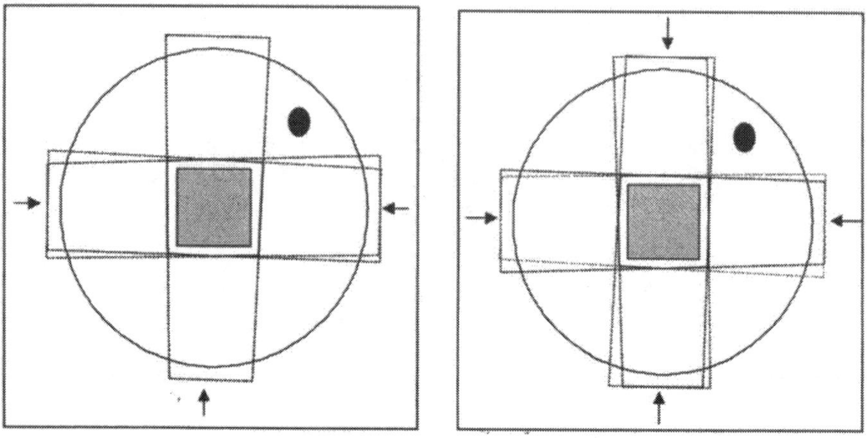

5.5 a) Three field plan 5.5 b) Four field plan

Fig. 5.5 Illustrating the ability of the geometrical approach to reproduce traditional beam settings for Plan 5.1

Ability to Account for OARs in Standard Plans. When the irradiation of an OAR is unavoidable, the treatment planner ensures that a low dose is delivered to the OAR by maximising the distance between the beam entry point and the OAR, thus enabling the radiation to be attenuated by the body structures. In order to demonstrate the ability of the algorithm to either avoid irradiating the OAR or at least give rise to a potentially minimised dose to the OAR, a plan, subsequently referred to as Plan 5.2, involving a circular body contour and circular PTA and OARs is used. The aim is to produce the best match between the PTA and the RBO whilst at the same time ensuring that the beam entry points are as distant from the OAR as possible. With a circular OAR, the best beam orientation involves equispaced beams. When use is made of five equispaced beams, it is not possible to avoid the OAR, see Fig. 5.6a. However, it can be observed, that, according to the prerequisites, the beams overlaying the OAR have their entry points closer to the PTA than to the OAR. This confirms the findings in [139] where a solution was selected to ensure that only one beam irradiates the OAR.

If it is required to avoid delivering any dose to the OAR, then it is necessary to change the preferences of the DM which selects solutions from the Pareto optimal set *a posteriori*. The solution shown in Fig. 5.6b is chosen to spare completely the OAR with the minimal possible cost for the PTA.

It is interesting to note, in Fig. 5.6b, that the beams close to the OAR have their beam entry points closer to the OAR than to the PTA. This provides the means to achieve a better match between the RBO and the PTA.

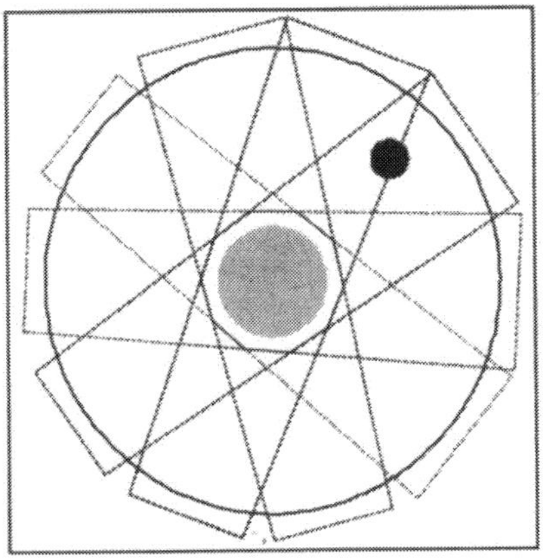

5.6 a) Minimum cost in the PTA for a low cost in the OAR (Equispaced beam paths)

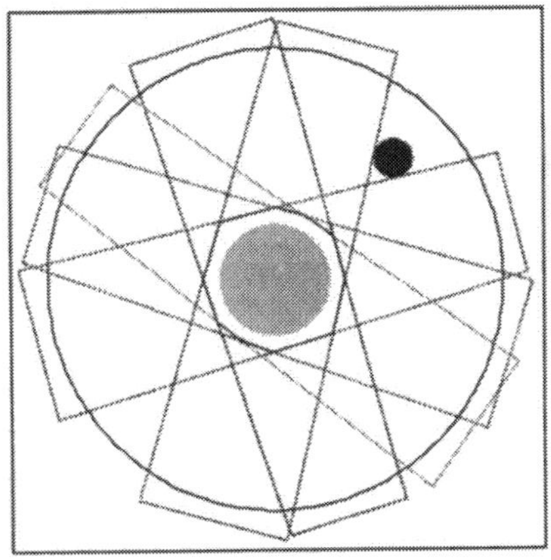

5.6 b) Minimum cost in the PTA provided cost in the OAR is null (Non equispaced beams)

Fig. 5.6 Illustrating effect of the OAR on the beam orientation and entry point for Plan 5.2

Note also that in Fig. 5.6a all the beam entry points are located in the same half plane. This is due to the fact that the cost in the OHT is not taken into account in the selection of the solutions resented in Fig 5.6. This may result in an undesirable unbalanced plan with dose much higher in the region close to the beam entry points. In order to prevent this a rotation of 180° amongst the neighbouring beams is required. This observation prompts the need for an additional operator which could add or subtract 180° to alternate the beams whilst taking into account the relative priorities of the OARs and the PTA.

Ability to Produce Beam Settings for IMRT Plans. When planning IMRT treatment it is necessary to take into account the ability of the beams to be modulated such that a specific portion of the beam facing an OAR can be attenuated. In order to assess the ability of the modified formulation, see Sect. 5.4.4, to account for the use of intensity modulated beams a plan, subsequently referred to as Plan 5.3, similar to that used in [140] is used. It involves a 'C' shaped PTA with an OAR within its concavity, see Fig. 5.7. The position of three beams is optimised with respect to C_{OAR} and C_{PTA}, see Sect. 5.4.4 using both the original, see Fig. 5.7a and the modified formulation, see Fig. 5.7b. The original objective formulation produces a plan widely accepted involving a three field brick, with an anterior beam and two parallel opposed beams. The modified formulation leads to a plan involving two parallel opposed beams with a posterior beam. This is due to the fact that when the centre of the OAR is closer to the beam entry than the isocentre, the beam is split. This simulate the sparing of the OAR resulting from the modulation in intensity of the posterior beam. The latter demonstrated that the modified formulation lead to results which are in agreement with that of Stein *et al* [140].

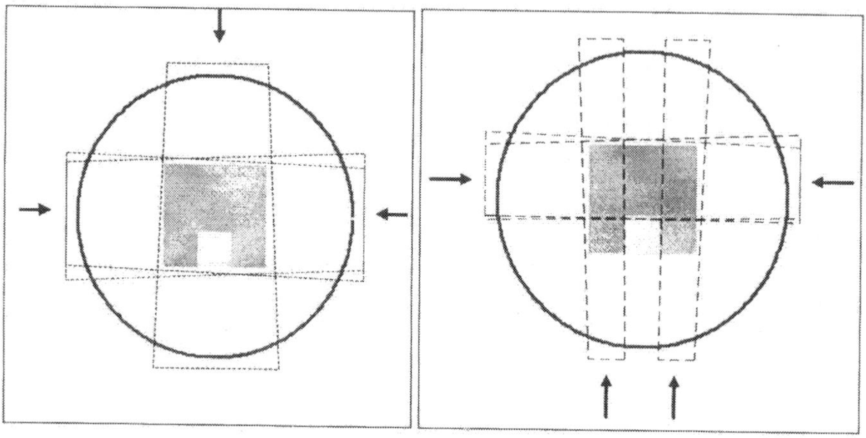

5.7 a) Traditional objective formulation 5.7 b) Modified objective formulation

Fig. 5.7 Comparison between the optimal beam arrangements produced using the traditional formulation and that generated by the modified geometrical formulation for Plan 5.3

Exploitation of the Pareto Optimal Formulation. In order to demonstrate the usefulness of the Pareto optimal approach use is made of Plan 5.4 for which optimal solutions can be selected by making use of *a posteriori* articulation of the objectives to fulfil different goals. Figure 5.8 shows the Pareto optimal set resulting from multiple runs of a MOGA with different articulation of the objectives (see Sect. 5.3). The objectives represented are related to the PTA and the OAR for 3, 4 or 5 beams. In order to illustrate the type of solution lying on the Pareto optimal set, four possible solutions have been selected. Three solutions were chosen such that the RBO fits as well as possible to the PTA, with little consideration being given to the OARs (the DM attempts to minimise only C_{PTA}). These solutions involved three five and four beams, represented in Fig. 5.8 by '+', 'x' and '*' respectively, with the corresponding beam paths shown in Fig, 5.9a, 5.9b and 5.10a, respectively. The last solution, which was chosen to enable a good sparing of the OAR, is represented by '⊕' in Fig. 5.8. The resulting beam paths, presented in Fig. 5.10b, shows that the RBO is much larger than the PTA.

It is interesting to note that from a geometrical view point there is little difference between the solutions chosen, so that C_{PTA} is minimal for 3, 4 or 5 beams. Indeed it is possible to conform to the PTA quite accurately with only three beams. This shows that in this case the minimal number of beams to conform to the PTA is three.

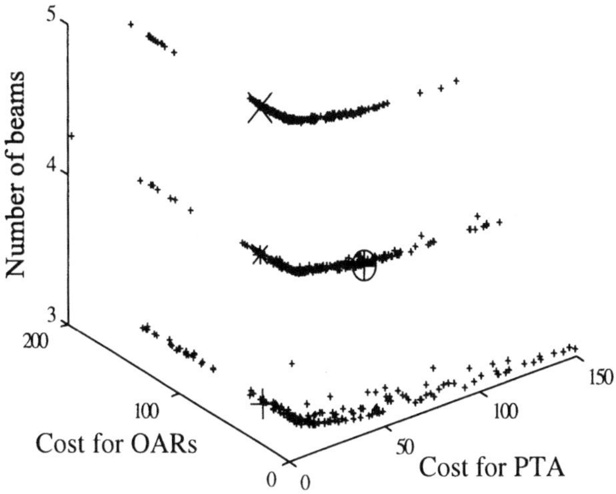

Fig. 5.8 Pareto optimal set (Plan 5.4) obtained by combining result form the optimisation of a MOGA with different fitness function; four solutions are selected from the Pareto optimal set represented by '×', '*', '+', and '⊕'

It can also be observed that C_{OAR} increases with the number of beams. This reflects the fact that more beams overlay the OAR. However this observation, made on a geometrical basis, may not always be confirmed by the assessment of the plans according to dose criteria. Indeed, provided that intensity modulation is used, the increase in the number of beams is generally followed by a diminution of the maximal dose received by the OAR, although a larger portion of the OAR might receive a dose.

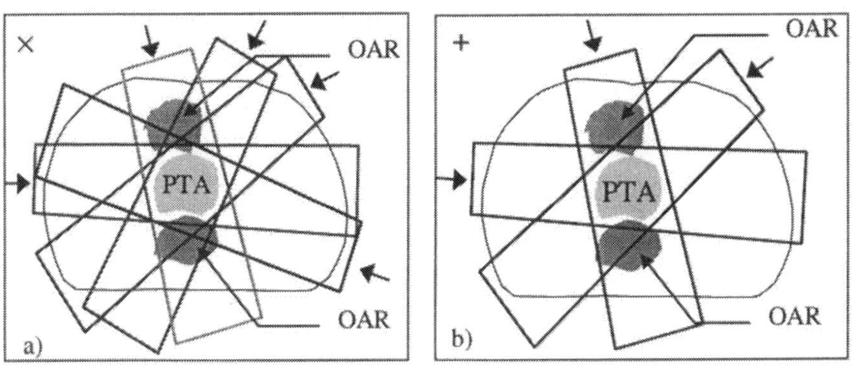

Fig. 5.9 Optimised beam orientation selected from Pareto optimal set (Plan 5.4) for a five field treatment plan represented by '×' in Fig. 5.8 and a three field treatment plan represented by '+' in Fig. 5.8

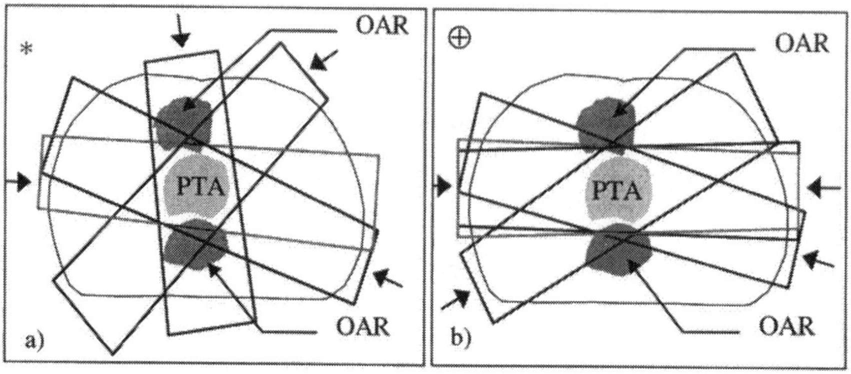

Fig. 5.10 Optimised beam orientation selected from Pareto optimal set (Plan 5.4) for a four field treatment plans with a high degree of conformation to the PTA, represented by '*' in Fig. 5.8, and another four field plan selected for its low cost C_{OAR}, represented by '⊕' in Fig. 5.8

It is interesting to note that the three beam plan forms the basis of the five and four field plans shown in Fig. 5.9a and 5.10a respectively. Indeed all these plans involve very similar gantry angles for three of their beams. This is mainly due to the use of the first problem specific operator described in Sect. 5.4.6).

Nature of the Solution Space. In order to investigate the effect of a particular treatment prescription on the solution space, and therefore emphasise the importance of the Pareto optimal approach to reach all the regions of the solution space, four different treatment plans are considered, namely Plan 5.1, Plan 5.2, Plan 5.4 and Plan 5.5. Two objectives are considered, namely minimising the cost for the PTA and thc OAR for three up to five beams.

Figure 5.11, shows the solution space resulting from Plan 5.1. It is only composed of three solutions, with all the solutions being able to completely fulfil the second objective, i.e. to minimise the cost for the OAR. It can be observed from Fig. 5.11 that there is little difference in the cost for the PTA between the solutions for three and four beams, and even less between four and five beams. Considering other objectives involving the area covered in the OHT would show that the maximum number of beams required for this plan is four. In this case, if a weighted sum were to be used at the beginning of the optimisation, only the cost for the PTA would be required to be taken into consideration.

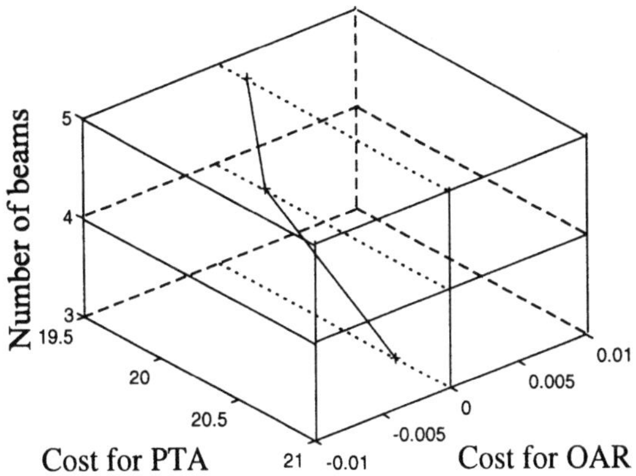

Fig. 5.11 Illustrating the solution space for Plan 5.1 involving a square PTA

The solution space for Plan 5.2 shown in Fig. 5.12, illustrates another notable effect, namely the improvement of the dose distribution with an increase in the number of beams. Such improvements, however, become negligible as the number of beams increase above five, especially when IMRT is used [140, 141]. This can be accompanied by an increase in the cost for the OAR, when a more and more accurate match is attempted between the PTA and the RBO.

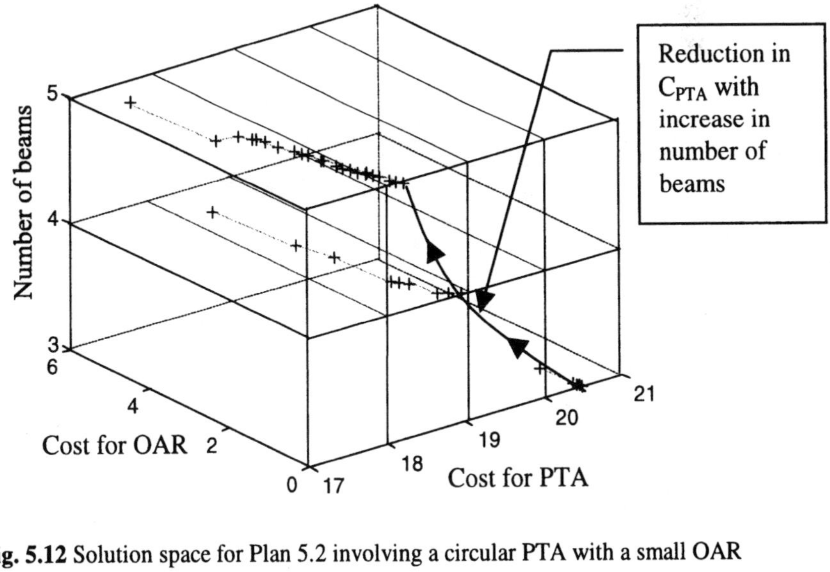

Fig. 5.12 Solution space for Plan 5.2 involving a circular PTA with a small OAR

Note that although only a marginal improvement can be achieved by increasing the cost associated with the OAR for the three beam case, increasing the number of beams leads to a more substantial improvement of the cost for the PTA with respect to the cost achievable with a sparing of the OAR. The conflict between minimising the cost in the PTA and the cost in the OAR becomes apparent.

Plan 5.5, for which the solution space is shown in Fig. 5.13, illustrates the occurrence of concave regions in the solution space. These regions cannot be attained when use is made of a weighted sum approach. Indeed, this is one of the advantage of the Pareto optimal approach, in that *a posteriori* solutions may be chosen anywhere on the Pareto optimal set. Examples of solutions obtained from the Pareto optimal set are shown in Fig. 5.14.

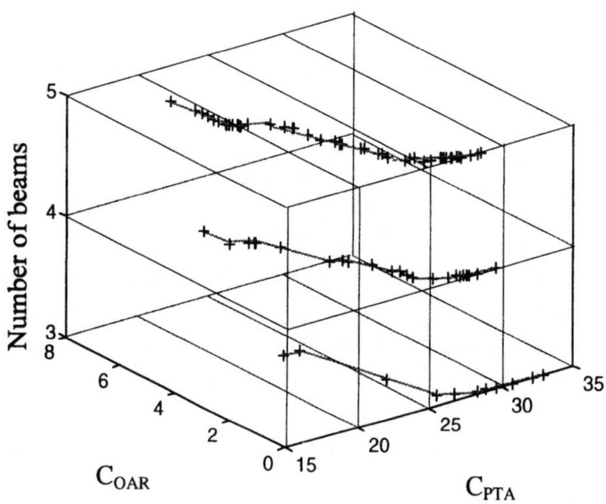

Fig. 5.13 Illustrating pareto optimal sets (Plan 5.5) for three, four and five beams

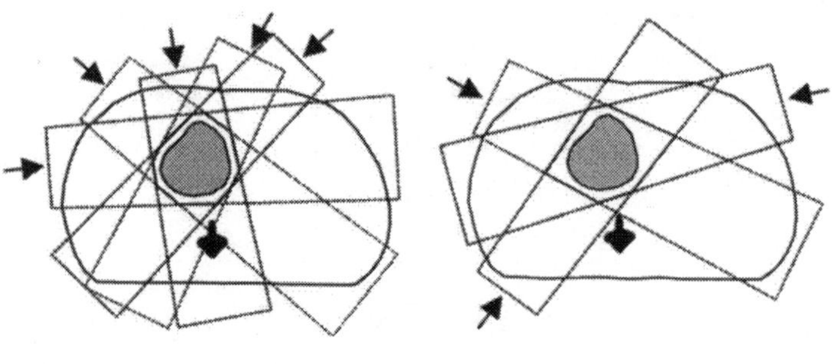

Fig. 5.14 Examples of solutions lying on the Pareto optimal set for Plan 5.5

5.4.8 Influence of Optimal Beam Orientation on Dose Distribution

To assess the benefits of the coplanar beam orientation achieved using the geometrical approach, use is made of a typical transverse computed tomography (CT) slice in the pelvic region, first represented in Fig. 1.8 and referred to as Plan 5.6. The beam orientation is optimised, using a MOGA with progressive articulation of the objectives, for three, four and five fields treatment plans. In addition to the number of beams, six regions of interest are considered: the PTA, the OARs, including the rectum, the spine, the left and the right femoral heads, with all the other structures grouped into the OHT category. The value of the objectives, or costs, for each ROI is calculated using both traditional and modified formulations. The normalised costs are represented in Fig. 5.15.

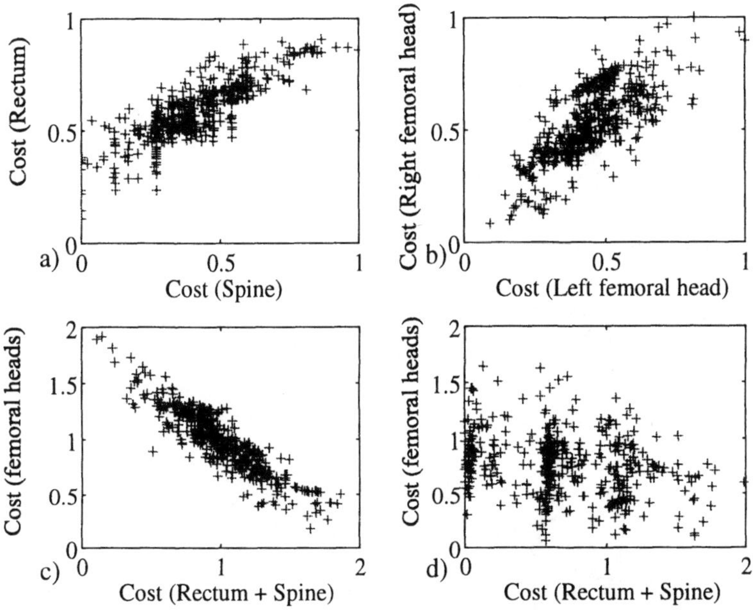

Fig. 5.15 Illustrating the use of the Pareto optimal formulation (Plan 5.6) to determine objectives correlation and compare traditional with modified formulation of the objectives

The cost for the spine was plotted against the cost for the rectum, see Fig. 5.15a, and the cost for the right femoral head was plotted against the cost for the left femoral head, see Fig. 5.15b. In both cases the plotted solutions indicate that a degree of correlation exists for the objectives describing the spine and the rectum as well as the right and the left femoral heads. Because there is no beam path which avoids both the group comprising rectum and spine and the group composed of the left and the right femoral heads, a low cost cannot be achieved simultaneously for both groups, using the conventional approach, see Fig. 5.15c. When use is made of the modified approach, however, it would appear that it is possible to achieve a low cost for both group of ROI see Fig. 5.15d. This would imply that the degree of inverse proportionality between these two regions is reduced when use is made of the modified formulation.

The optimisation algorithm was run several times with both the traditional and the modified formulation and the resulting solutions grouped together. Three candidate solutions were selected from the solution set using a goal attainment method and subsequently compared to solutions involving a three field brick, a four field brick and five equispaced beams. The goal for each objective O_i was expressed as:

$$C_{Oi}^2 \Big/ \max(C_{Oi}^2) < x_i \tag{5.16}$$

where the x_i are values chosen experimentally to be 1.35, 30.00, 30.00, 40.00, 40.00 and 18.00 for the PTA, the spine, the rectum, the right left femoral head, the left femoral head and OHT respectively (in the case of a five beam plan). Different values for the x_i are chosen for the case of three and four field plans, noting that as the number of beams decreases, the values of x_i associated with the PTA increases. To fully justify the geometrical approach, the plans selected using the geometrical objectives for three, four and five beams, see Fig. 5.16 and 5.17, are subsequently optimised according to dose criteria, using a method based on adaptive weighted least squares, described in Chap. 4. The resulting dose distributions, shown in Fig. 5.18 and 5.19, are normalised such that the mean dose delivered to the PTA is 100%.

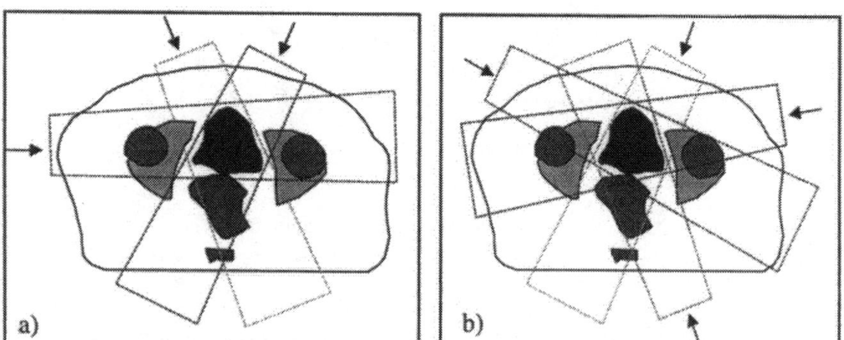

Fig. 5.16 Optimal beam path (Plan 5.6) for a three and a four field plan using traditional objective formulation

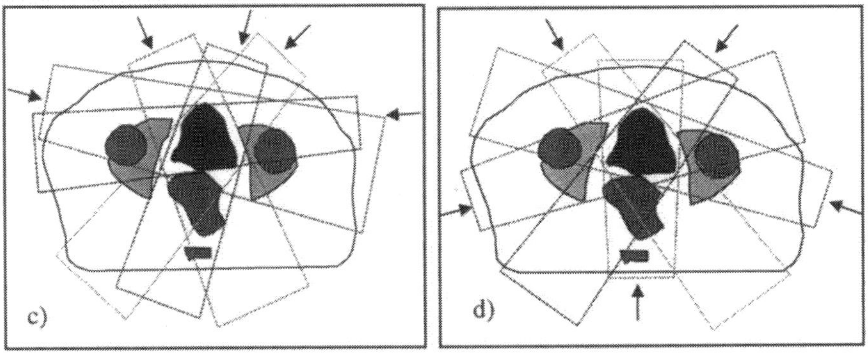

Fig. 5.17 Comparison between optimal beam path (Plan 5.6) for a five field plan obtained using traditional objective formulation and five equispaced beam selected in accordance with the findings in [139, 140]

In all cases it can be observed that the shape of the area where all the beam overlap is very similar to the shape of the PTA. This ensures that the high dose region conform well to the PTA, see Fig. 5.18 and 5.19. The dose in the OHT is also very similar, however, as expected, the three field plan which irradiates a larger volume with a higher dose. In all cases the rectum receives a maximum dose below 40%, and an average dose below 30%, which is considered satisfactory. The femoral heads receive a maximum dose below 60% and a mean dose below 45%, with the lowest dose received by the femoral heads being delivered using the three field treatment plan.

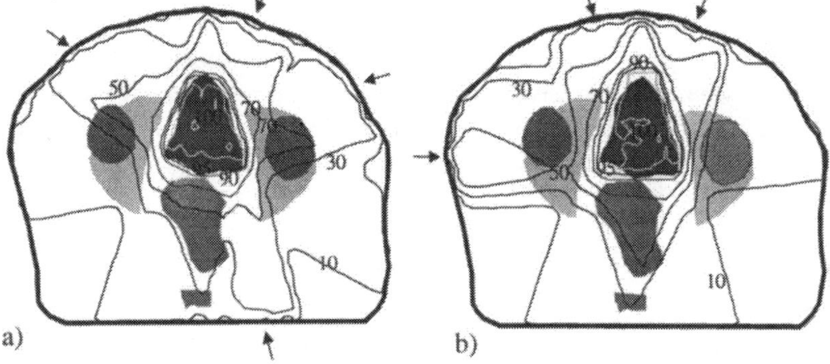

Fig. 5.18 Dose distribution obtained for optimised beam orientation and IMB for Plan 5.6

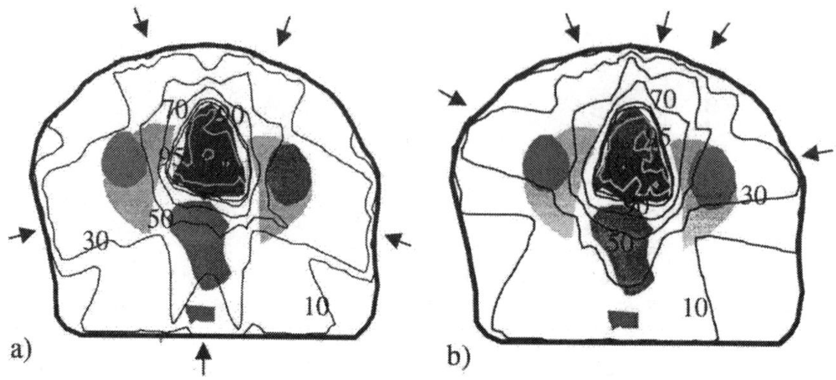

Fig. 5.19 Illustrating isodose contour plots (Plan 5.6) for standard beam orientation and optimised IMB

It can be observed from Fig. 5.18 that there is little difference between the five fields plans, see [139]. This confirmed the findings of Stein *et al* [140] and Söderström and Brahme [141].

To demonstrate the dose improvement made possible by the optimisation of the beam orientation when a small number of intensity modualted beams are involved, consideration is given to four field plan. The dose area/volume histograms given in Fig. 5.20, show that the four field brick is worse than the four field optimised plan, represented in Fig. 5.16b and 5.18a, except in the PTA region. In this case optimising the position of the beams results in improvements for all the OARs and OHT. The improvement is particularly noticeable on the integral dose area histograms for the rectum, the femoral heads and the OHT, where the curve, represented by '–•' , is much lower than the curve represented by '-'. This confirms previous observations in [28, 139] where optimisation of the a three field plan gives rise to improved dose distributions. Increasing the number of beams results in a further improvement of the dose distribution as well as the degree of conformation in the PTA.

Remark: Note that the fact that optimised beam orientation give rise to improved distribution is not surprising, however, traditional beam arrangements are still widely used in conjunction with wedges due to their simplicity of implementation and to the fact that the outcome of such techniques are well documented. Further, making use of a four field brick may irradiate a relatively large amount of OHT, but as the PTA may move and evolve during the course of treatment it is considered as a safe option ensuring that the cancer is eradicated.

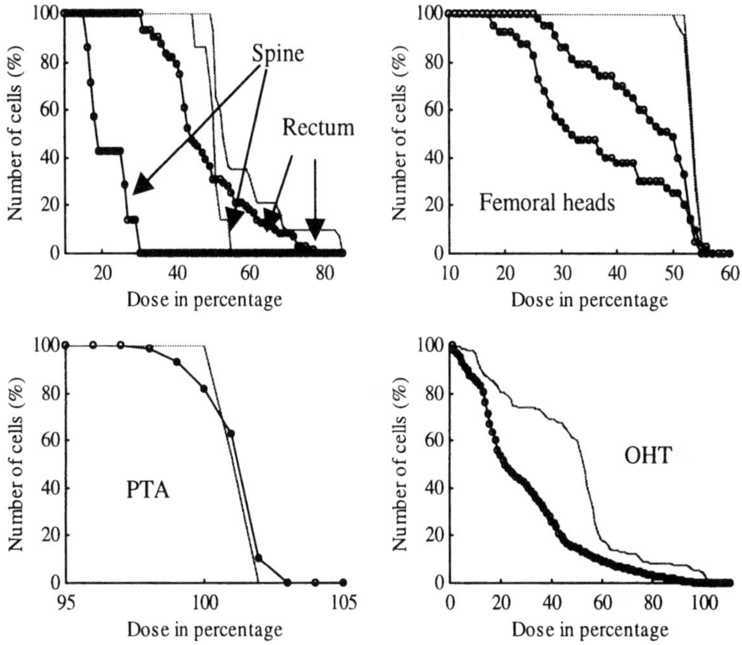

Fig. 5.20 Integral dose area histograms (Plan 5.6) illustrating advantages of geometrically optimised beam orientation, represented by -o- , compared to standard four field brick, represented by '-'

5.5 Optimisation of Beam Weights and Wedge Angles

Traditional radiotherapy makes use of wedges to shape the beams, with such an approach being optimised manually, given the relatively small number of fixed wedges available (see Chap. 1). However, the introduction of more modern techniques, making use of universal wedges have increased the number of wedge angles available to the clinician and physicists to plan their treatments. Universal wedges of nominal angle $\theta_w = 60°$ can be used to produce any effective wedge angle θ_E, between $0°$ and θ_w by treating a patient for part of each fraction with the universal wedge field, and for the other part of the fraction with an open field (i.e. where no compensating material is inserted into the beam path). In [86], an exact relationship between the so called effective wedge angle θ_E and the nominal wedge angle θ_w has been derived, but in the context of treatment plan optimisation, the following simplified expression proposed by Philips Medical Systems Division (1983) [143], is widely used:

$$B = \tan \theta_E / \tan \theta_w \qquad (5.17)$$

where B is the weighting of the fraction of the wedged field, that is combined with the fraction (1-B) of an open field to give the nominal wedge angle θ_E. However, there are various other techniques available to produce wedged fields, therefore, in this work, in order to present a solution that does not depend on the practical implementation, each beam is represented by one beam weight and one wedge angle. The resulting wedged beam may then be produced using traditional static techniques combining an open field and a wedge, or dynamic technique making use of MLCs.

The increased versatility due to the number of possible beam wedge angles results in an increase in the complexity of the problem perceived by the treatment planner to determine the optimum beam weightings and wedge angles. As a consequence, automation of this time consuming task has been identified as an area where significant benefit can be made and this forms the main objective of the work detailed in this section.

5.5.1 Brief Review of Existing Techniques

The number of variables being small compared to the inverse problem and the beam dose distribution being calculated in a rapid manner have led to the domination of heuristic search techniques that are much simpler to implement than traditional calculus based inversion techniques. In this context, SA has been used successfully in [4, 37] to determine the optimal beam weight combination. However the high computational effort required by traditional SA makes it a slow process which was considered unrealistic for use in RTP systems. In order to overcome this problem, fast SA (FSA) has been applied [36, 37, 87] and it has been shown to converge up to ten times faster than standard SA. Constrained SA [88] has also been used to find a feasible solution for a set of constrained beam weights. The constraints can be modified so that if early convergence occurs, the set of constraints is relaxed, i.e. the minimum beam weights are reduced so that a new possible solution can be attained. In addition, random optimisation with non-linear score fit and constraints (RONSC) [89, 90] has been developed to determine a feasible solution for objective functions based either on physical or biological constraints.

Sherouse [144] proposed a mathematical method, based on a vector relationship, which enables the selection of wedge angles, wedge orientation and beam weight in 3-D for homogeneous media. Each beam is represented by a dose vector perpendicular to the isodose surface. The method aims to combine these vectors (one per beam) such that their sum is null at the isocentre of the target region. A null gradient ensures that the dose over the target is homogeneous. The approach provides a useful conceptual basis, but it is limited to simple shapes and therefore may not be able to provide solutions for the wedge angle and beam weight optimisation problem, especially for inhomogeneous media and complex target shapes. More recently GAs have been used for beam weight optimisation and favourably compared to SA [92]. However the published work concerning applications of GAs in RTP is still very much in its infancy.

5.5.2 Coding Strategies

In [126] it has been shown that the use of problem specific operators could slightly improve the performances of a MOGA dedicated to the optimisation of beam weight and wedge angles. However, these improvements are not considered as significant. This is due to the fact that the operators have been designed to replicate current practice of manual optimisation, however, the latter may not all be desirable (i.e. non optimal).

In this section use of binary coding with traditional GA operators is described, with consideration being given to the optimisation of wedge angles and beam weights for a treatment plan involving two fields (i.e. four unknown elements), where each chromosome represents a combination of wedge angle and beam weight.

Coding of the Beam Weights. The beam weightings characterise the strength of the beam. In order to avoid hot spots (or high intensity dosage) at least three beams are normally used to treat cancer in the pelvic region. This ensures that each beam weighting is less than 100%, i.e. the dose at equilibrium is less than the dose received by the PTA. In this work, the beam weight is assumed to vary between 0% and 100% with a precision of 1% being required, hence, an alphabet A = 101 is used to code each beam weight. Making use of binary coding seven bits are required to represent integer values constrained in the interval [0,127]. Note that the beam weights are often in the range [30% 60%], and therefore in most cases six bits could be sufficient to code the beam weight. However in order to produce plans that require beam weightings outside this range one more bit is added.

Coding of the Wedge Angles. The wedge angle is the physical angle between the normal to the CAX and a line tangential to the isodose curve at a depth of 10 cm [64], (see Chap. 1). It is physically represented by an integer constrained in the range [-60, 60] and can also be coded with seven bits.

Each beam weight and wedge angle is therefore represented by seven bits. When use is made of binary coded GAs, each individual is a vector of integers representing two beam weights and two wedge angles. Each chromosome, being the overall coded representation of these beam weights and wedge angles, is 28 bits long, i.e. 14 bits per beam. The relationship between the physical variables and the coded variables is given in Table 5.2.

Table 5.2 Relation between coded representation and physical meaning of the variables involved in beam weight and wedge angles optimisation

Variable	Beam weight	Wedge angle	Beam weight	Wedge angle
Physical value	23%	0°	68%	-30°
Coding system	binary	binary	binary	binary
Genotype	0010111	1000000	1000100	1100000
Phenotype	23	0	68	-30
Chromosome	0 0 1 0 1 1 1 1 0 0 0 0 0 0 1 0 0 0 1 0 0 1 1 0 0 0 0 0			

5.5.3 Simulation Studies

In order to demonstrate the capabilities of the MOGA to optimise beam weights and wedge angles, use is made of Plan 5.6. This plan is relatively complex as an OAR is adjacent to the PTA, however it is still realisable as the PTA is convex. Indeed in [1, 126] it has been shown that a prescription involving concave PTA could not be physically achieved with the use of a limited number of wedged beams. This is an important consideration when issuing a treatment plans. Note, however, that in [88] it has been shown that slightly concave distributions could be achieved with wedges, provided that a large number of beams can be used. However, such a large number of beams is not a clinically viable solution, therefore in this work it is preferred to make use of a few conformal fields for concave PTA, leaving the use of wedges to convex PTA.

It has been seen that several strategies can be adopted to orientate the search to a particular region of the Pareto optimal set. In this work it is believed that use can be made of a DM based on the weighted sum approach with an adaptive error weighting similar to that developed in Chap. 4. Such a DM should direct the search algorithm to a region that is likely to offer a good trade-off solution.

Optimising Objectives Independently. Three objectives are considered for the optimisation, and each is expressed in a quadratic form such that sum of the square of the error between predicted and prescribed dose is minimised. In order to focus the attention of the algorithm, a dead band like action is used (see Chap. 4), where errors corresponding to dose points within specification are set to zero. Such an action may result in dose distribution that lacks uniformity in the PTA when used in conjunction with ILS. However, the use of compensators as beam shaping devices produce inherently smooth distributions, therefore this procedure is considered to be appropriate.

Making use of such an approach it was observed that the corresponding 'best solution', according to the DM, was not lying on the Pareto optimal set. This may seem surprising as a weighted sum approach would result in a solution that is non dominated. However, the accuracy of the dose within the PTA was taken into consideration by the DM whereas it was not directly optimised. (This is due to the dead-band action within the cost associated with the PTA.) Note, however, that it is still possible to select a Pareto optimal solution by making use of another DM usually based on preferences, and therefore acting much more like a human to select an appropriate solution. In order to overcome this apparent problem the original DM was modified to account for the dead-band like action. Making use of such an approach it can be observed, see Fig. 5.20, that the solutions selected by the DM are now appropriately lying on the Pareto set, thus highlighting the benefits of the Pareto optimal approach in the design of a clinically appropriate DM.

Exploitation of the Pareto Optimal Formulation of the Objectives. Once that the Pareto optimal set has been obtained it is necessary to select the most appropriate solution. This solution may not be the one favoured by the DM that was used to guide the search, in this case a new DM procedure has to take place. In fact the most interesting feature associated with *a-posteriori* articulation of the objectives is that it is possible to chose a solution which is the most suited for a particular individual. Fig. 5.21 shows solutions lying on the Pareto optimal set that results from a multiple run of a MOGA with various DM (see Sect. 5.2 and 5.3).

It is interesting to note that all the solutions shown in Fig. 5.21 do not belong to the Pareto optimal set, which reflects the fact that some rank differentiation methods are better than others in finding non dominated solutions. It has been observed during the simulations that the most robust approach is that of randomly alternating the objectives used to differentiate between the non dominated solutions (see Sect. 5.3.2).

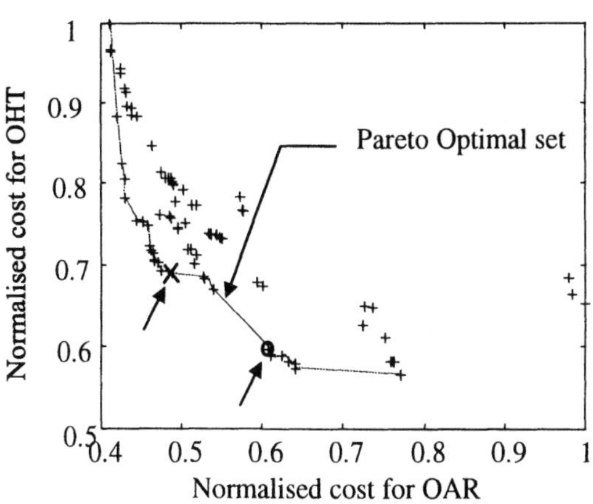

Fig. 5.21 Illustrating the selection of two candidate solutions lying on the Pareto optimal set

Two solutions have been selected from the Pareto optimal set of Fig. 5.21. The first solution, represented by a '×' for which the isodose plot is shown in Fig. 5.22, is chosen to produce a relatively low error in the OARs whilst keeping the error in the OHT at a reasonable level. However, the isodose plot reveals that although the sparing of the OAR is acceptable, the plan is unbalanced, with the right side of the plan receiving a dose 10% higher than the left side. In order to compensate for this effect creating hot spot, a new solution was chosen, indicated by a 'o' in Fig. 5.21. The isodose plot, see Fig. 5.23, shows that the hot spot on the right side of the plan has been removed, at the expense, however, of a higher dose delivered to the OARs, with two thirds of the OARs receiving a dose of at least 30%. Such a dose level is, however, still acceptable. It is interesting to note that the use of a Pareto optimal approach overcomes the difficulties reported in [36, 37] where the optimised plans were relatively likely to be unbalanced with unacceptable hot spots.

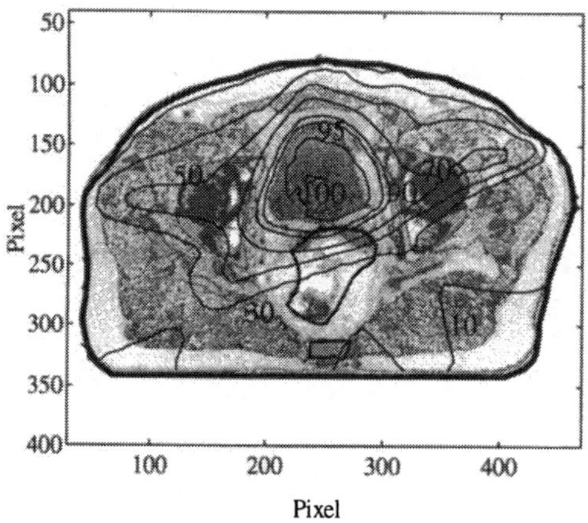

Fig. 5.22 Illustrating the isodose plots (Plan 5.6) obtained for a solution, represented by '×' in Fig. 5.21, chosen for its relatively low dose delivered to the OARs

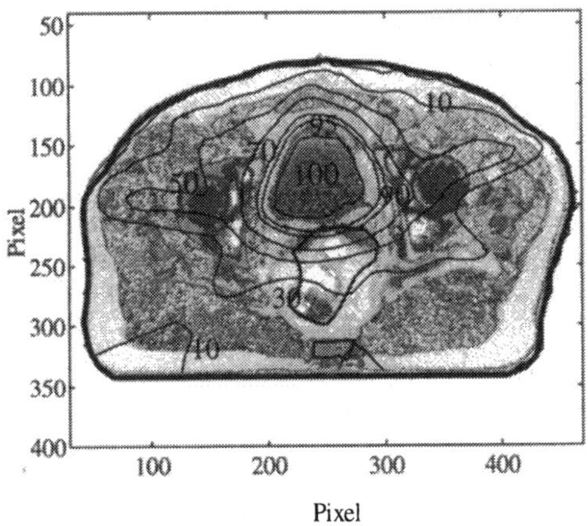

Fig. 5.23 Illustrating the isodose plots (Plan 5.6) obtained for a solution, represented by 'o' in Fig. 5.20, chosen for its relatively low error in OHT resulting in the equalisation of hot spots

Remarks: For both solutions a highly accurate dose is achieved in the PTA, however the OHT in the neighbourhood of the PTA were also affected by a high dose. By comparison with the dose distribution obtained with intensity modulation, smoother dose distributions are obtained with wedges with a smaller dose gradient on the edges of the PTA. This is due to the fact that the effect of the penumbra is no longer accounted for in the optimisation process and, in order to cover all the PTA, it is necessary to ensure that the penumbra region is outside the PTA. This leads to an overdosing of the tissues on the edge of the PTA. For simple case like this with convex PTA shapes, correcting only for the effect of the penumbra could improve the degree of conformation significantly.

5.6 Concluding Remarks

This Chapter has presented a novel approach to optimisation in RTP involving a heuristic technique, namely a multi-objective genetic algorithm, aimed at solving multiple-objectives in parallel. This approach leads to the determination of a family of solutions, as opposed to a single solution, lying on the Pareto optimal set. The Pareto optimal approach enables the clinician to search in parallel for solutions and to emphasise either the sparing of OARs or achieving a high and homogeneous dose over the PTA. It enables changes in the preference of the DM *a-posteriori* to ensure, for example, that the plan selected is not unbalanced.

A hybrid MOGA has been used to solve the coplanar beam orientation in a transverse plane. It has been shown that the proposed geometrical formulation of the objective is able to replicate the behaviour of more traditional formulations based on dose requirements. Indeed it has been shown that the beam orientation chosen on geometrical basis gives rise to an improved dose distribution over a standard beam arrangement. It has been shown in [126] that hybridising a GA can improved its overall performance. The use of the Pareto optimal approach has highlighted the difference that exists between the treatment plans with respect to the degree of correlation of the objectives. Such a formulation should potentially enable adaptation of the objective to the type of treatment plan.

A more traditional binary coded MOGA has also used to solve for beam weights and wedge angles. It has been shown that the Pareto optimal formulation could be useful in the design of cost functions and DMs as it offers the possibility of assessing the compromised solution selected by the DM to the overall set of non dominated solutions.

CHAPTER 6
EXPERIMENTAL VERIFICATION OF OVERALL APPROACH

6.1 Introduction

The purpose of this Chap. is to provide an experimental verification of the approach as well as to give a technical summary of the various aspects involved in the practical implementation of beam intensity modulation via patient specific compensators. By drawing on the RTP optimisation techniques presented in the previous Chap., the remaining practical procedures involved in the determination of optimal intensity modulated beams (IMBs), and hence compensator profiles, a fully integrated RTP procedure is demonstrated. It is the culmination and the combination of all these techniques that has made possible the prediction, optimisation and, for the first time in the UK, the verification and realisation of conformal radiotherapy with in field intensity modulation on a demanding, yet realistic test case.

The overall proposed approach, that should in turn lead to the automatic generation of a fully optimised RTP system with the production of optimal patient specific compensators, has been assessed under clinical conditions on a torso phantom. A realistic test case designed for the purpose of the experiment attempts to simulate the most demanding treatment for cancer located in the pelvic region, such as prostate cancer. The geometry of the ROIs is such that a treatment plan that irradiates all the PTA whilst, at the same time, sparing the OARs and the OHT could not be achieved with standard beam compensation techniques. In fact the PTA is concave in nature, with part of the OAR being enclosed by the concavity.

By adopting a step by step approach, the Chapter presents the various steps involved in the optimisation of a RTP. Similar to current practice, the procedure starts by making use of a coplanar beam orientation scheme introduced in Chap. 5 to determine the optimal beam orientation. This is followed by an approach that combines and adapts the heuristic and deterministic search techniques presented in Chap. 4 and 5 to the IMB optimisation problem in the form of a two-stage hybrid technique. In the initial stage, use is made of iterative least squares (ILS), together with the parallel beam model developed in Chap. 2 and 3, to solve the inverse problem and determine a 'theoretical' solution. This solution is used to generate an initial population that can then be evolved by a multi-objective genetic algorithm (MOGA) combined with a Pareto optimal approach with progressive articulation of the objectives (see Chap. 5). The use of this heuristic optimisation technique enables the search space around the trade-off solution found with ILS to be enlarged. It has the additional advantage of being able to make use of a more realistic divergent beam model to solve for the optimum set of IMB in a forward manner to produce a physically realisable IMB profile.

The optimised compensator profiles are then deduced from the IMB profiles making use of an iterative technique. Attenuation within the compensators is modelled using an exponential function to account for the primary attenuation coupled, with a point spread function to account for scatter in the compensators.

The overall approach is assessed using both radiosensitive film and a radiosensitive gel dosimeter. Film is a well tried media to record variation in radiation intensity enabling the assessment of the relative dose distribution. Whilst gel dosimeters are still very much in their experimental phase of development, they are now recognised as providing an ideal means of validating dose distributions. The results are encouraging and indicate a good agreement between predicted optimised dose and that actually achieved.

6.2 Optimisation of Conformal Radiotherapy Treatment

A Combination of Techniques. Whereas in the previous Chapters the various aspects of optimisation of RTP were introduced, this section focuses attention towards the ultimate combination of the techniques detailed in the previous Chapters from the beam modelling stage to the use of novel heuristic techniques to solve for the coplanar beam orientation problem and finally the determination of optimised IMBs.

Whereas the beam orientation is determined with the same geometrical technique as has been detailed in Chap. 5, the optimisation of IMBs requires some refinements to be incorporated within the optimisation procedures based on the ILS approach presented in Chap. 4. Essentially, the ILS scheme made use of a simplified parallel beam model to determine optimal solutions quickly (in 10 to 50 iterations). However, the quality of the resulting optimal solution depends on the appropriateness of the *a-priori* selection of the objective weightings associated with the quadratic cost function. In Chap. 5 it was shown that the Pareto optimal approach, implemented via a MOGA, to the optimisation of beam weight and wedge angle could overcome the problems linked to *a-priori* selection of a compromised solution by selecting the most appropriate solution *a-posteriori*. However, this approach, which requires a more thorough investigation of the solution space, is more computationally intensive. In order to 'speed up' the overall optimisation, a hybrid scheme has been developed which aims to combine the desirable features of both analytical ILS and random search MOGA techniques whilst reducing their respective drawbacks (see Table 6.1). ILS is used to determine a good initial solution in only a few iterations whilst the MOGA is used to adapt the solution obtained with a parallel beam model to a more complex divergent beam model whilst introducing an additional degree of freedom in the type of objective function used. By doing so, the lengthy initial stage of the optimisation, requiring the determination of a likely region of the solution space, is much reduced as ILS produces a good initial solution. The MOGA can then extend the search around the region pre-selected by the ILS scheme.

The other important aspect of realising IMB, is to ensure that the solution predicted is physically achievable. Therefore, the inherent limitations imposed on the gradient of neighbouring IMBs (or pencil beams) by the beam modulator (i.e. compensator) are required to be accounted for. The latter, However, was not directly taken into consideration in the prediction stage and constitutes an area of identified further work.

Table 6.1 Comparison between analytical (ILS) and heuristic (MOGA) procedures

	ILS	MOGA
Beam model	Problem specific model designed to solve the inverse problem	Any beam model expressing a relationship between IMB and dose distribution
Objectives	Quadratic formulation involving a weighted sum of the objectives	Any form: linear, non-linear, objectives considered independently
Solution (s)	A single solution that minimise a trade-off objective function	A set of non dominated solutions
Selection of the optimal solution	Weighted sum of the objectives	Use of a DM that can use preference, goals, or weighted sum of objectives
Optimality	local optima	local optima or global optima
Speed of convergence	10 to 100 iterations	100s to 1000s iterations

Algorithmic representation of the overall hybrid procedure involved in issuing a dose prediction.

i) Issue a dose prescription (see Sect. 6.4)

ii) Optimise the coplanar beam orientation with a MOGA (see Chap. 5, Sect. 5.4)
iii) Select an acceptable solution from the Pareto optimal set
iv) Determine an initial solution with ILS and parallel beam model (see Chap. 4) from the optimal beam setting obtained in iii)
v) Map the original solution obtained with a parallel beam model onto a divergent beam model (may introduce some error if the number of IMBs is not identical)
vi) Generate an initial population for the MOGA by modifying the initial solution with small random variation and keeping the solution obtained in v)
vii) Run the MOGA with a divergent beam model to determine Pareto optimal solutions
viii) Use a DM to select the most appropriate solution from the Pareto optimal set
ix) Determine the compensator profile from the IMB profile (see Sect. 6.3)
x) Deduce a tool path for the CNC machine used to manufacture the compensators (see Sect. 6.3)
xi) Assess the resulting dose distribution (see Sect. 6.4).

The various aspects involved in steps ii) to step viii) have previously been dealt with in Chap. 4 and 5, and will not be repeated. The only difference between the MOGA used to optimise the beam weight and wedge angles and the one used to optimise IMB is that in the latter a real number representation is used [11, 126]. Recall that use of real numbers removes the coding and decoding stages of the procedure and allows the use of genetic search operators designed for real coded GAs, such as for example intermediate recombination and discrete mutation [28, 126, 139]. The various intermediate results leading to the prediction of a dose are dealt with in Sect. 6.4, whereas the procedures concerned with the modelling and manufacture of the compensators are dealt with in the Sect. 6.3.

6.3 Modulating Beam Intensity with Compensators

6.3.1 Compensator Preliminaries

The pencil beam model developed in Chap. 2 and 3 provides a relationship between the beam profile **b**, which is proportional to the dose at the point of equilibrium $\mathbf{d}_{max}$, and the beam dose distribution **d**. The introduction of a compensator into the beam path affects the radiation emitted from the source and therefore the dose observed at x_{max}. In Chap. 3, it has been shown that the pencil beam model developed is able to replicate conformal dose distributions provided that the correct beam profile is used as an input to the 'beam' system. However, the model does not take into consideration the effect of attenuating material outside the body structures. It is therefore necessary to establish such a relationship to be able to model the effect of the compensator on the dose distribution. Having already established a relationship between the dose distribution and the beam profile, it is now only necessary to determine a relationship between the beam profile and the compensator thickness. The two-stage process used to determine the dose distribution from the IMB profile and the compensator profile is illustrated in Fig. 6.1.

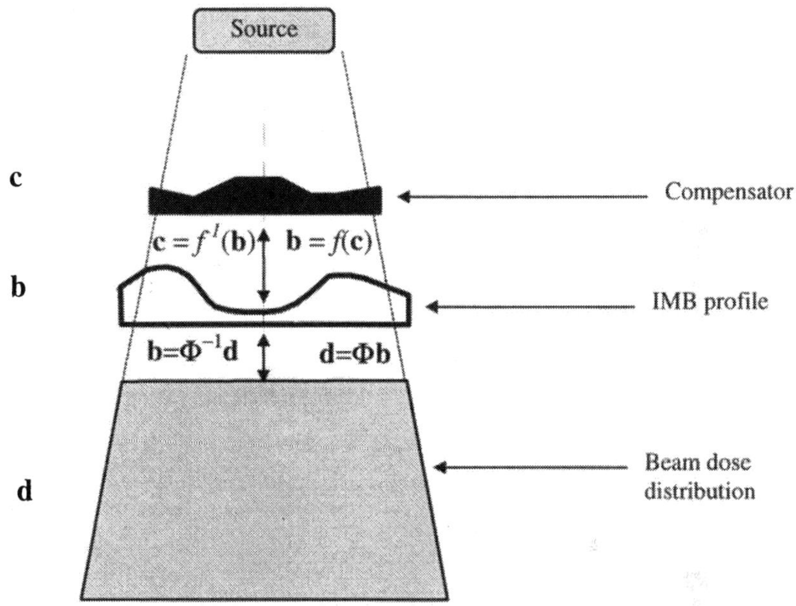

Fig. 6.1 Illustrating the approach used to model the interaction of radiation in the compensator independently to the interaction of the radiation within the body structures

The compensators used in this work are manufactured in a low melting point alloy, namely MCP 200 [145], which is a tin-zinc alloy with a density of 7.10^3 kg/m^3. This particular alloy has been chosen because it offers an interesting compromise between a dense material such as lead or low density material such as wax which are of similar density to the human body structures. Indeed, for dense materials small thickness variation may be marked by significant dose attenuation which, given the means used to form the compensators, may be undesirable. Conversely low density materials require a significant thickness to attenuate the radiation. Traditionally wax materials are used to compensate for uneven patient contours, whereas, the increased ability of the dense material, such as MCP 200, to attenuate radiation make it an ideal material to modulate beam intensities. Another advantage of MCP 200 is that its low melting temperature makes it a reusable resource. As such once a particular compensator is obsolete, it can be melted down and re-used to produce a new compensator. This is of particular importance for hospitals where resources are limited.

6.3.2 Modelling of the Compensators

The effect of compensators on radiation is similar to that of the human body structure in that it attenuates radiation as an exponential function of the compensator thickness. The attenuation p due to the compensator, expressed in % is defined as follows:

$$p = 100\, e^{-\mu c} \tag{6.1}$$

where c is the compensator thickness and μ is a linear attenuation coefficient.

Making use of equation (6.1), the thickness (or height) of the compensator is given by:

$$c = \frac{1}{\mu} \ln\left(\frac{D_{\%}}{100}\right) \tag{6.2}$$

where $D_{\%}$ denotes the IMB profile and is the calculated %DD at the point of equilibrium.

Making use of this relationship to deduce a compensator profile from the IMB profile would result in producing a compensator profile that is the mirror image of the IMB profile. The resulting dose measured from such a compensator would result in a smoother profile than expected due to the effect of scatter within the compensator. In order to include the non negligible scattering effect within the compensator an additional term is added to the primary component. This is achieved by making use of a point spread convolution function [1, 119].

This point spread function is then convoluted with the primary compensator profile calculated from equation (6.1). The beam profile used to generate the tool path in the manufacture of the compensator can then be identified by iteratively modifying the elemental compensator thickness to achieve the best match between the required profile and the profile resulting from the convolution of the primary attenuation by the point spread convolution function.

In order to assess the benefits of conformal radiotherapy via compensators, a five field treatment plan was devised, see Sect. 6.4.1. It involves the manufacture of five compensators from blocks of MCP 200, see Section 6.3.3. Prior to the manufacture of these compensators, the 'ideal' (i.e. assuming that the compensator profile produced can actually be manufactured) compensator profiles have to be calculated from the IMB profiles. All the compensators involved in the experiment have been determined using a two stage approach, which is fully described in [1]. It involves:

- Determining a first estimate of the compensator profile by making use of equation (6.2)

- Iteratively refining the first estimate of the compensator profile in an attempt to replicate the desired IMB profile

6.3.3 Manufacture of the Compensators

The compensators are manufactured with an industrial standard computer numerically controlled (CNC) machine and tool path generating code. In order to cut a MCP 200 block, it is necessary to feed the CNC machine with the correct tool path. This tool path is deduced from the compensator profile which is itself obtained from the IMB profile. The path generated is the path followed by a vertical axis orthogonal to the surface and passing through the centre of the cutting tool head. With the cutting tool used to produce the compensators being 6 mm in diameter, it is necessary to offset the tool path by half of this diameter, i.e. 3 mm. The CNC tool path code generator used in this work is only capable of accounting for an offset of the tool in one direction, whereas in order to be able to manufacture a compensator with a minimum of handling, it is necessary to offset the cutting tool in two directions. As a consequence, the offset of the cutting tool had to be calculated manually. In order to illustrate the approach, a 'W' shaped compensator profile is considered, see Fig. 6.2.

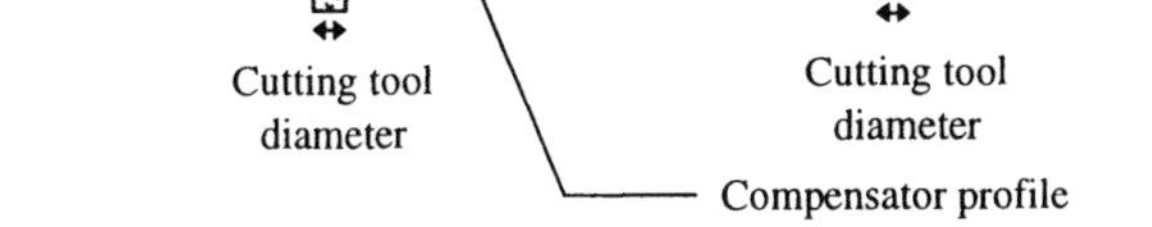

Fig. 6.2 Illustrating the generation of a tool path from a 'W' shaped compensator profile

Note the offset of the tool path in both left and right direction. Due to the cutting tool characteristic, it is not possible to produce a sharp edge at the bottom of the 'valleys'. This can result in a small over/underestimation of the attenuation depending on the strategy adopted to calculate the tool path.

Once the tool path has been generated, MCP 200 can be melted down and moulded into a cubic block which can then be cut by the CNC machine to produce the required compensator, see Fig. 6.3 showing the compensators manufactured in Walsgrave Hospital NHS Trust.

The profiles used to create the tool path, accounting for the cutting tool characteristics, for the five compensators used in the field trial are represented in Fig. 6.4, 6.5, 6.6 6.7 and 6.8.

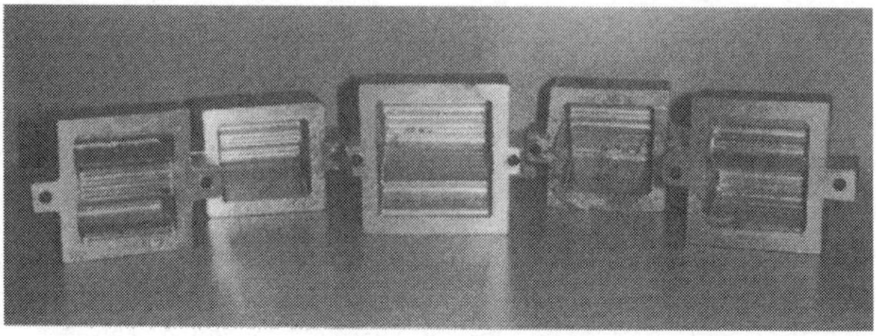

Fig. 6.3 Illustrating the five compensators that were used in the experiment and manufactured by a CNC machine at Walsgrave Hospital NHS Trust, Coventry

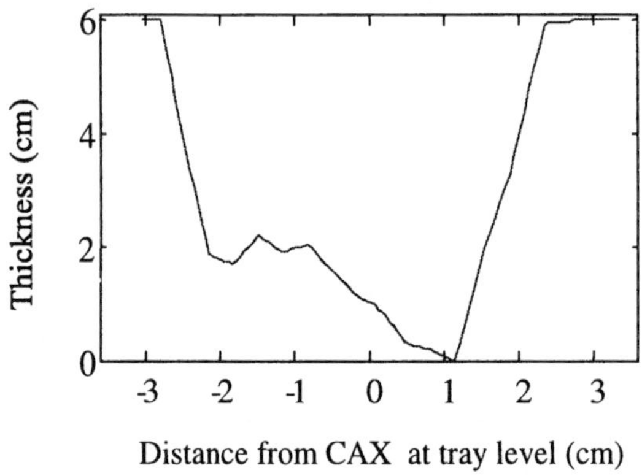

Fig. 6.4 Compensator profile for beam 1 including the correction for the tool path

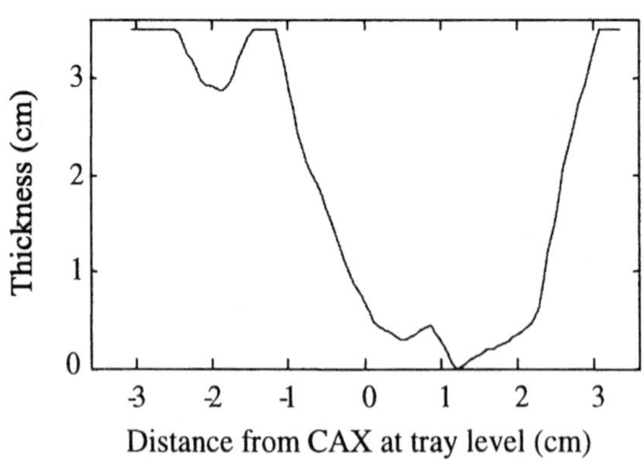

Fig. 6.5 Compensator profile for beam 2 including the correction for the tool path

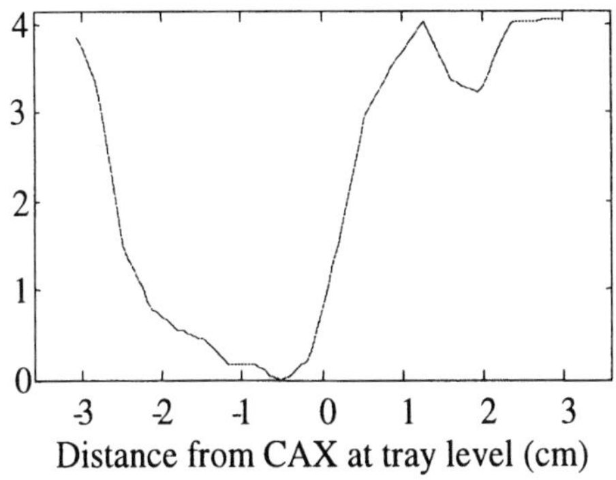

Fig. 6.6 Compensator profile for beam 3 including the correction for the tool path

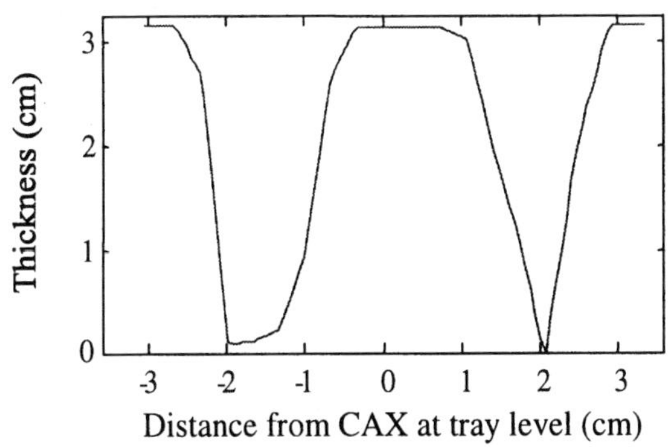

Fig. 6.7 Compensator profile for beam 4 including the correction for the tool path

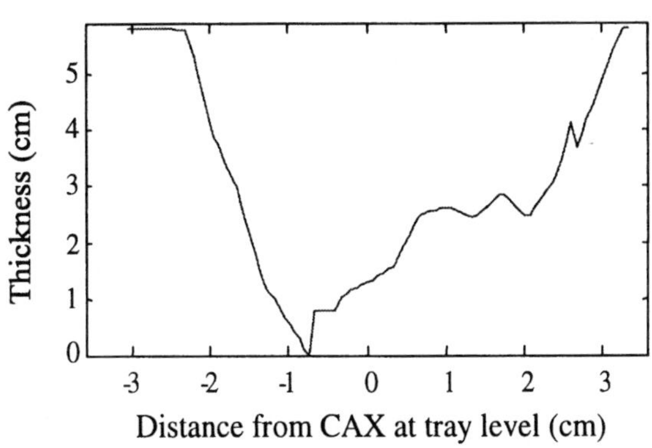

Fig. 6.8 Compensator profile for beam 5 including the correction for the tool path

6.3.4 Determination of the Number of Monitor Units

In radiotherapy, prescriptions are given in terms of dose in Gray (Gy) (J/kg) or centiGray (cGy) received at the isocentre, that is usually located in the middle of the cancerous region or PTA. Radiotherapy treatments are usually delivered in a number of fractions, each fraction corresponding to a given irradiation time, thus a given portion of the total dose. The treatment machines that are used to deliver these doses are calibrated under specific test conditions, which are easily reproducible. A full field ionisation chamber* is placed directly in the radiation beam adjacent to the source. It monitors the amount of radiation passing from the source by collecting the charge produced. The amount of charge collected is referred to as the number of monitor units and has no absolute physical value. The charge collection is altered such that one monitor unit corresponds to a given dose. In Walsgrave Hospital, linacs are calibrated with respect to a 10 cm by 10 cm field with a SSD equal to 100 cm, see Fig. 6.9. Under these conditions, one monitor unit correspond to a dose of 1 cGy. Note that the distance from the source to the point of dose measurement (at depth x_{max}) is at SSD + x_{max} from the source.

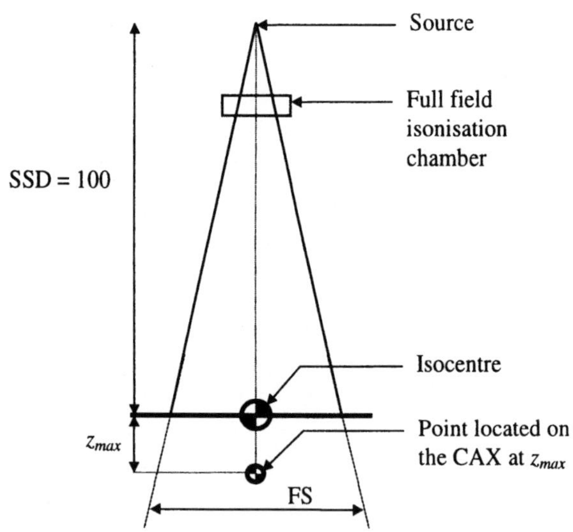

Fig. 6.9 Reference setting for the beam under calibration condition, i.e. 10 cm × 10 cm open field at 100 cm SSD

The practical delivery of the radiation in the experimental trials involved the determination of the number of monitor units for each of the intensity modulated

---

* A full field ionisation chamber is an ionisation chamber that encompasses all of the beam.

beams involved in the treatment plan. In order to achieve this, it was necessary to measure the output factor of each compensator with respect to the calibration conditions, see Fig. 6.10.

The measurement procedure involved the location of the compensator at its exact location on the tray, with use being made of the same field size as in the prescription, and was offset if necessary, see Fig. 6.10. The linac was then set to deliver 100 monitor units (mu) and the dose actually measured at the point of equilibrium was recorded. Table 6.2 shows the dose recorded for a 25 MV linac.

Table 6.2 Output factors for the modulated field used in the experimental verification

Compensators	beam 1	beam 2	beam 3	beam 4		beam 5
Dose in Gy measured at x_{max}	0.617	0.555	0.81	0.638	0.560	0.706

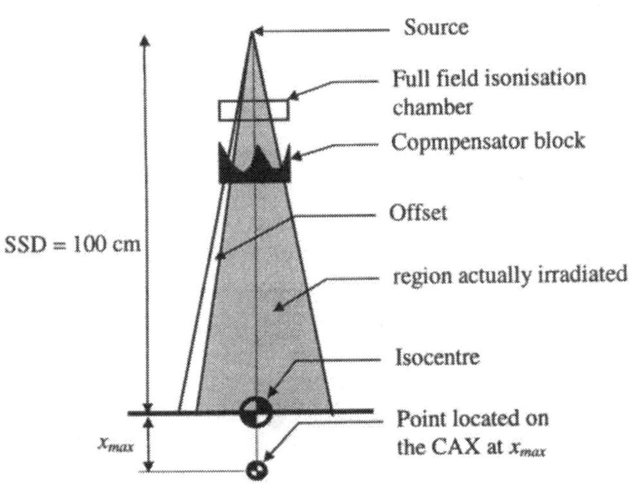

Fig 6.10 Accepted practice to determine the output factor for a compensated/ blocked field

Note that the dose measured is less than 1 cGy due to the presence of the compensator combined with the use of a smaller field size than the field size used for calibration. Note also that beam 4 is delivered in two fractions. This was due to the fact that with the thickness of the compensator being limited, the attenuation in the middle of the field was not sufficient, creating an undesirable overdosage. In order to solve this problem, the field was divided into two smaller fields that were delivered sequentially.

These measurements enabled the determination of the number of monitor units, with respect to the calibration conditions, that was required to deliver a dose of 1 Gy. However, all the measurements were performed under a different setting than that used in the actual delivery of the treatment, see Fig. 6.11.

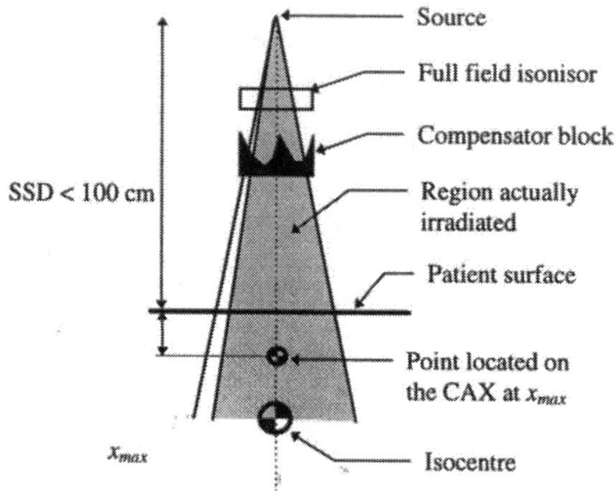

Fig. 6.11 Set up used during the delivery of the treatment

It can be observed from Fig. 6.11 that the SSD is now less than 100 cm. This is due to the fact that in order to simplify the delivery of the treatment, the linac is usually rotated around the patient about the isocentre. The isocentre is generally situated at the middle of the cancerous region or PTA, with the source to the isocentre distance being 100 cm. As a consequence, the SSD varied with the beam orientation and a correction factor was required to be introduced for each compensator that was calculated assuming 100 cm SSD. The attenuation of radiation in the air being proportional to the square of the distance, see Chap. 3, the number of monitor units needed to be modified by the ratio R of the square of the distance between the SSD for each beam and the SSD used for calibration, such as:

$$R = \frac{SSD_i^{\ 2}}{SSD_{ISO}^{\ 2}} \tag{6.3}$$

where SSD_{ISO} is the source to skin distance for the calibration condition, or the source to isocentre under experimental conditions; SSD_i, i=1...N_{beam} are the SSDs for each of the beams obtained by subtracting the distance from the isocentre to the patient surface to SSD_{ISO}. The ratio R are given in Table 6.3.

These measurements combined with the dose prescription, enabled the calculation of the number of monitor units to be set for each beam involved in the experiment. The number of monitor units M_i calculated with respect to the calibration condition is given by

$$M_i = \frac{D_i}{o_i \left(\frac{100}{SSD}\right)^2 c} \tag{6.4}$$

$$\text{where } D_i = D_{ISO} \frac{T_i}{T_{ISO}} \tag{6.5}$$

where D_i corresponds to doses at the point of equilibrium (3.5 cm depth for 25 MV), T_i corresponds to the numerical value at the same point in the predicted isodose distribution and o_i are the output factors of the compensators given in Table 6.4. The subscript *ISO* refers to the point of intersection of all the beams, which is a single point known as the isocentre. In the first experiment D_{ISO} = 60 cGy, T_{ISO} = 100, with the predicted percentage depth dose T_i, i=1...5 and the number of monitor units given in Table 6.4.

Table 6.3 Ratios used to account for the difference between the SSD used for the calibration and the SSD for each of the beam involved in the treatment

Compensators	beam 1	beam 2	beam 3	beam 4	beam 5
Ratio used to correct for SSD	0.689	0.656	0.723	0.792	0.774

Table 6.4 Predicted percentage depth dose at x_{max} and corresponding number of monitor units for a 25 MV photon beam used at Walsgrave Hospital NHS Trust, Coventry

Compensators	beam 1	beam 2	beam 3	beam 4		beam 5
Percentage depth dose T_i	53.9	52.0	40.0	34.0	34.0	49.8
Output factor o	0.617	0.555	0.705	0.638	0.560	0.706
Number of monitor unit M_i	32.0	31.0	18.0	19.0	21.0	27.0

Remark: The number of monitor units depend mainly on the thickness (or height) of the compensator on the central axis, where the dose is measured. This explains why identical percentage depth dose at x_{max} gives rise to a different number of monitor units.

6.3.5 Schematic Representation of the Overall Approach

The overall approach from the optimisation of a treatment plan for IMRT to the manufacture of patients specific compensators is illustrated in Fig. 6.12.

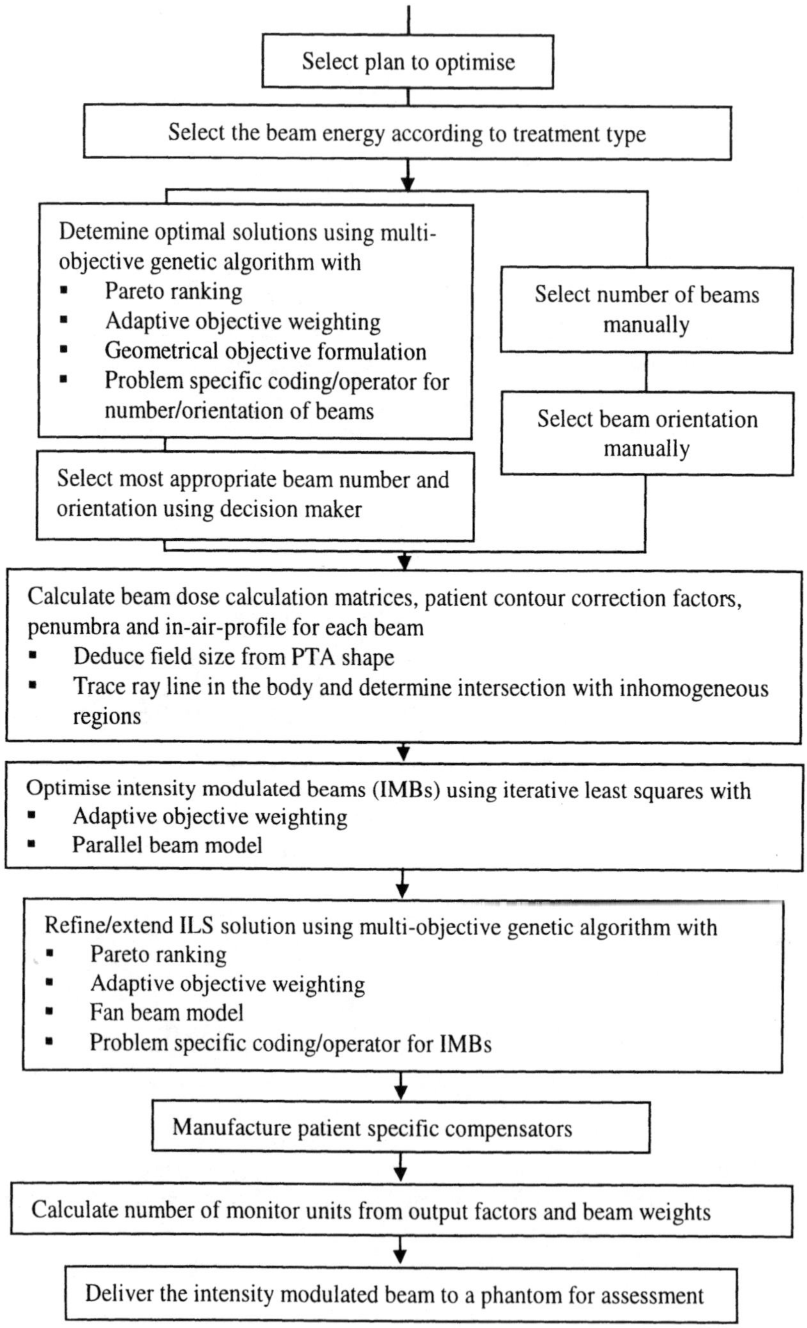

Fig. 6.12 Illustrating the overall approach from the selection/optimisation of number and orientation of beams to the optimisation of beam profiles and the delivery of treatment via patient specific compensators

6.4 Experimental Verification of Intensity Modulated Radiation Therapy

The aim of the experimental work was to demonstrate the capabilities of the overall strategy proposed to predict, optimise and realise beam intensity modulation with patient specific compensators. In order to do so it is necessary to assess the outcome of the conformal plan. At this stage of the work, however, such an assessment cannot be made on patients. Indeed, prior any acceptance of any new technique in the clinical environment, it is necessary to ensure that the technique is safe, and that the dose distribution predicted can be delivered accurately and consistently. Only once these prerequisites have been fulfilled can the benefit of a particular technique be assessed in clinical trials. In order to assess the reproducibility of the predicted dose distributions two different media were used. The first experiment involved the use of a radiosensitive film that is a well established media to record variation in dose intensity. The second method made use of a technique that is still in an experimental stage, known as gel dosimeter. The distribution obtained with the gel dosimeter was subsequently verified with a film positioned onto a custom designed film holder.

6.4.1 Assessing Dose Distribution with Film

Similar to visible light, ionising radiation affects photographic film such that it varies in the level of greyness, or density, according to the exposure with the shade of grey deepening as the exposure increases. For each film, the relationship between the exposure and the so called photographic density is characterised by its 'Hurter-Driffield' curve [1], see Fig. 6.13.

In radiotherapy, as the level of exposure to be recorded is high, 'slow' film is required to be used, i.e. film that reacts less quickly to exposure. In addition, in order to be able to differentiate exposure variation, it is necessary to ensure that the linear section of the Hurter-Driffield curve is used, i.e. above and below the levels for which optical density can be differentiated. In the experimental research work reported here, a slow film is irradiated by a maximum dose in the region 60 - 80 cGy. This ensures that it is possible to differentiate between dose levels in the target area. Note that the dose level of 60 cGy corresponds to 100%.

Once irradiated, such a film can be inspected visually to provide a reasonable overview of the dose distribution. However, due to the limitations of the human vision system, and in particular to its inability to differentiate between several different grey levels, such a visual inspection can be misleading. Therefore, in order to be able to assess density variation recorded by the film more accurately, use is made of a densitometer, where the output of the densitometer can be related to actual relative doses expressed in terms of percentage depth dose.

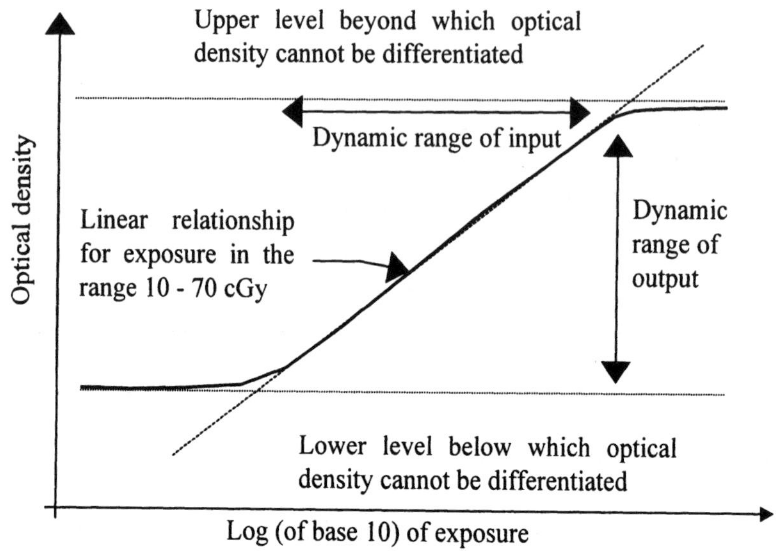

Fig. 6.13 Typical Hurter-Driffield curve for a slow film

Experimental Set-up for the Film. The set up for the film involves a three piece semi anatomical hardboard torso phantom used at Walsgrave Hospital for total body irradiation measurements. Hardboard is used as it offers a density similar to that of human body structures. The elliptical shape of the phantom attempts to emulate patient geometry in the pelvic region, see Fig. 6.14.

The phantom is set up exactly as a patient would be, with the slice containing the film inserted between the two other pieces of the phantom so that full 3-D scatter can be simulated. This arrangement means that the film represents a slice through a torso and therefore when it is exposed to the combination of intensity modulated beams produced by the compensators, it provides a density variation proportional to the dose received. Resulting two-dimensional dose distributions are then determined by scanning the film.

The compensators were fixed with two screws onto a perspex slider that was inserted into the tray fixed onto the head of the linac. All five metal compensators manufactured from the dose prediction were machined in the mechanical workshop of the Department of Clinical Physics and Bioengineering at Walsgrave Hospital NHS Trust, Coventry, as would be done with standard compensators.

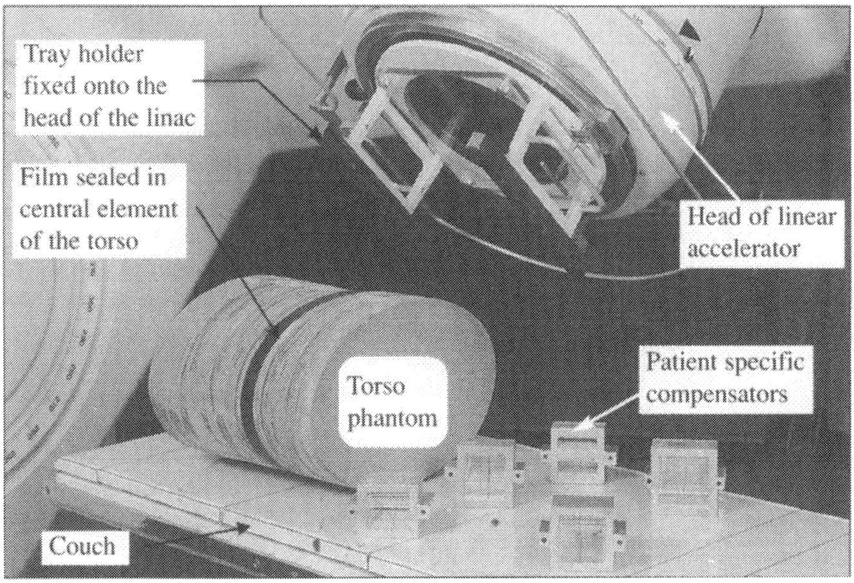

Fig. 6.14 Illustrating the equipment used to assess a five field conformal treatment plan with use being made of a film inserted into a torso phantom, courtesy of Walsgrave Hospital, NHS Trust, Coventry

Establishing a Dose Prescription. Making use of the torso phantom shown in Fig. 6.14, a demanding, yet realistic dose prescription was realised. The outline of the 'body' was measured to replicate the shape of a trans-axial slice of the torso phantom shown in Fig. 6.14. Several ROIs have been outlined to replicate anatomical structures encountered in the pelvic region, see Fig. 6.15.

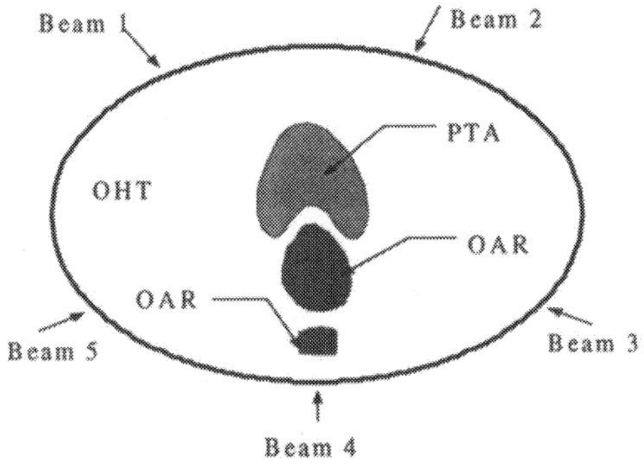

Fig. 6.15 Semi-anatomical torso phantom contour with ROIs outlined

The treatment plan involving a concave PTA, taken as being the prostate, was outlined such that the top of the PTA is similar to that of Plan 5.6, but with an OAR, taken as the rectum, in its concavity.

Selection of the Beam Orientation. The prescription required that a high dose be delivered in the PTA ($d_{PTA} = 100\%$) whilst a low dose be given to the rectum and a very low dose to the spine ($d_{OAR} < 20\%$). The beam orientation shown in Fig. 6.16, was originally selected using the traditional geometrical formulation, see Chap. 5, such that it conforms well to the PTA, with the limitation of the dose in the OARs being taken care of by optimising the IMB profiles. Note that the beam entry point of the posterior beam directly facing the spine was chosen manually (i.e. the original beam has been was rotated by 180°) to ensure that sufficient dose would be delivered to the branches of the PTA that are encompassing the rectum OAR.

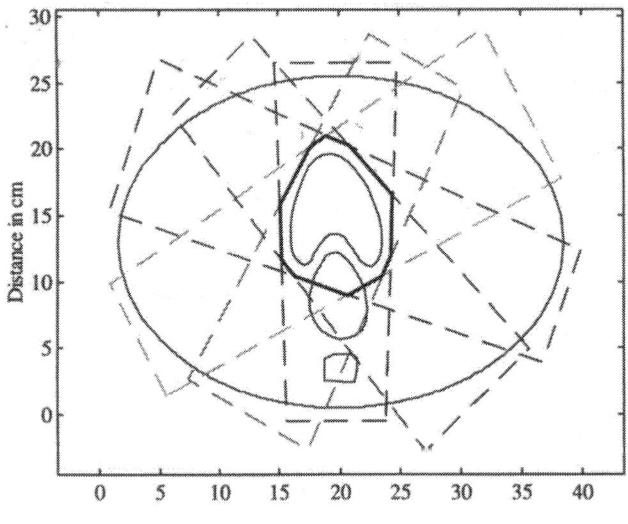

Fig. 6.16 Optimised beam orientation for semi anatomical torso phantom

Positioning of the Torso Phantom. The delivery of a conformal treatment required an accurate positioning of the compensators with respect to the patient. In order to do so, it was necessary to position the torso phantom such that each beam CAX passes through the isocentre of the PTA. This was achieved by making use of laser beams intersecting at the isocentre of the PTA, see Fig. 6.17.

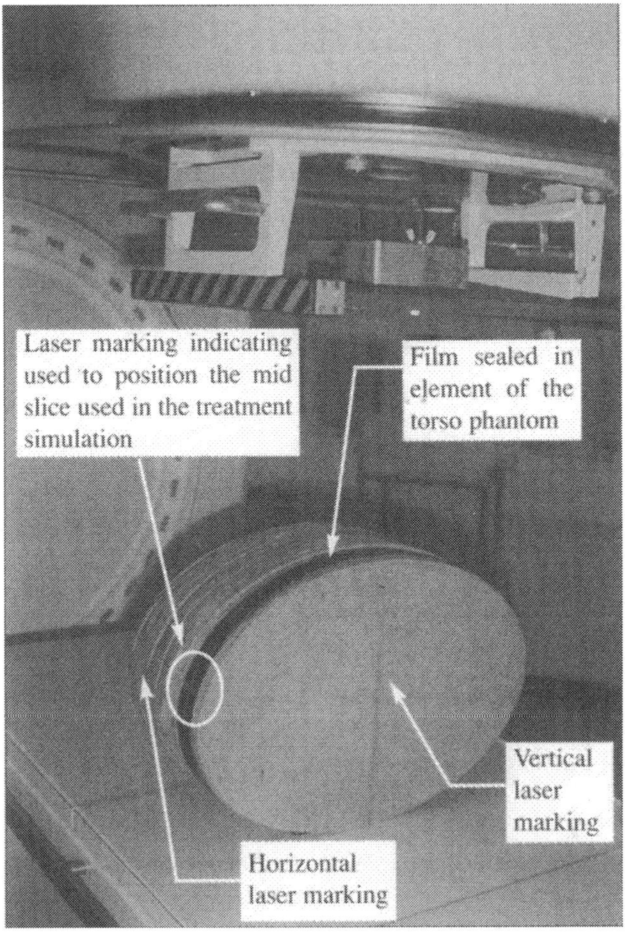

Fig. 6.17 Illustrating the use of laser markers to position the semi anatomical torso phantom accurately, courtesy of Walsgrave Hospital NHS Trust

Treatment Delivery Procedures. The radiation used to treat cancer is harmful for healthy human beings, and therefore it was necessary to take some precautions to ensure that the only subject/object receiving radiation is the patient or in the experimental test case the torso phantom. Treatment rooms are shielded to protect persons outside the room where the machine is located. Therefore, each time a dose fraction is delivered it is necessary to exit the treatment room. The procedures followed to deliver the six fractions necessary were as follows:

- Fix the compensator on the perspex insert onto the tray located under the head of the linac
- Position or reposition (when necessary) the torso phantom using laser marking

– Rotate the head of the linac according to prescription
– Select the field size with the appropriate offset
– Exit the room
– Fire the beam

Predicting a Dose Distribution with the ILS Scheme Developed in Chap. 4. The isodose plots shown in Fig. 6.18 have been calculated with use being made of the ILS routine developed in Chap. 4, together with a parallel beam model. The resulting IMBs represent a good first approximation of the beam profiles. The treatment plan issued shows a satisfactory coverage of the PTA whilst the OAR receive a dose around 30% for the rectum and less than 10% for the spine.

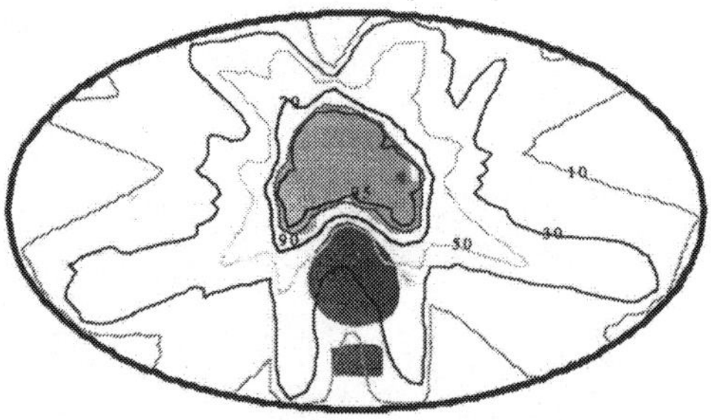

Fig. 6.18 Predicted isodose contour plot, for the hardboard torso phantom, with use being made of a parallel beam with ILS

Adapting the Prediction to a Divergent Beam Model with the MOGA Developed in Chap. 5. The IMB profiles obtained with a parallel beam model, are then adapted to a divergent beam model with a MOGA developed in Chap. 5. The resulting isodose plot is shown in Fig. 6.19.

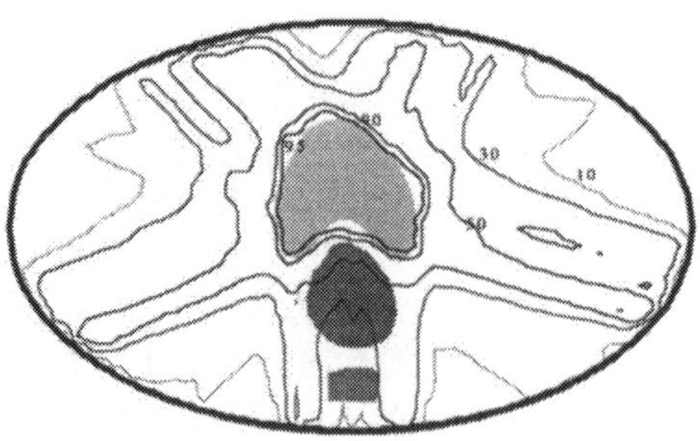

Fig. 6.19 Predicted isodose contour plot, for the hardboard torso phantom, with use being made of a divergent beam and MOGA

Note that the dose distribution adapted from the parallel beam used with ILS is not as good as the one shown in Fig. 6.18. This is due to the fact that the IMB resolution used with the divergent beam is not as high as the one used with the parallel beam. This is to reflect the fact that 'sharp' IMB variations are not achievable in practice.

Measuring the Actual Dose Distribution. Figure 6.20 illustrates the resulting dose distribution obtained with five 25 MV intensity modulated beams.

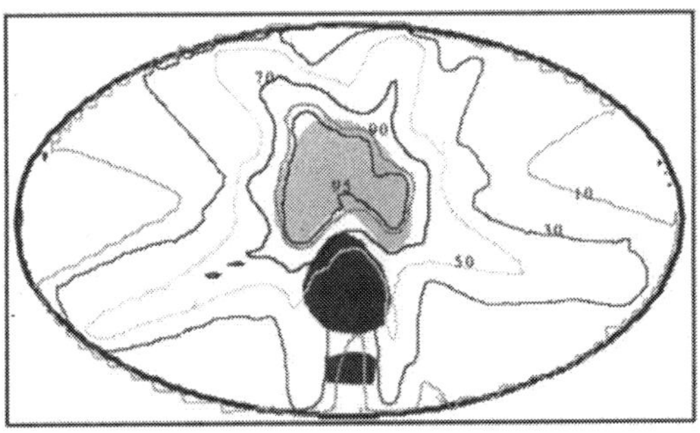

Fig. 6.20 Digitised isodose contour plot, for the hardboard torso phantom, obtained from the development of the film used to demonstrate the feasibility of conformal radiotherapy

It is interesting to note also that in Fig. 6.18, 6.19 and 6.20 the sparing of the OARs is clearly visible. A high dose region outside the PTA can be observed in Fig. 6.20 due to the over estimation of the beam weighting caused by the high gradient of the IMB profile about the central axis, which is emphasised again due to the relatively low resolution of the film, that is a direct result of the small number of units that can be delivered (only 60 cGy) [119].

In order to overcome the problems caused by the low resolution of the film, another technique making use of gel dosimeter has been used [146, 147, 148, 149], which, although still under experimental development, is now well recognised as providing an ideal means of validating dose distributions.

6.4.2 Assessment of Conformal Distribution with Gel Dosimeters

Gel dosimeters were proposed as early as 1966 [148], however, they have only recently become a practical and potentially extremely successful method for assessing dose distributions. This is due to the elaboration of a new gel composition [149] which overcomes the problems of post radiation diffusion previously encountered, which resulted in a poor spatial resolution of the gel. The gel dosimeter used in the experimental work carried out at Walsgrave Hospital

NHS Trust, Coventry, was developed at the Royal Leicester Infirmary, Leicester, UK [146, 147, 150]. The gel formed from bis-acrylamide-nitrogen and gelatine is termed BANG gel. The gel formulation used is based on that proposed by Maryanski in [145], and contains bis-acrylamide co-polymer (4%), polymer acrylamide (4%), gelatine (5%), with the nitrogen used to remove oxygen which inhibits polymerisation.

Radiation Induced Polymerisation. BANG gel works on the principle of radiation induced polymerisation [1, 119, 149]. Although the chemical processes involved in the underlying chemical mechanism are not yet fully understood, the basic principles involved in radiation induced polymerisation are as follows. By irradiating monomer molecules in the presence of cross linking agents, monomer molecules bind together and cross-link to form longer and more rigid molecules. The large size of these polymer molecules prevent them from diffusing through the gel matrix, which ensure a good spatial resolution. The dose distribution can then be deduced by making use of a magnetic resonance imaging (MRI) system to measure the so called relaxation rate (R_2) [150]. In the experimental work, the gel was imaged with an MRI scanner with a 1.0 Tesla magnet using a multi slice spin echo sequence. Since the polymerised molecules show a higher relaxivity in proportion to the absorbed dose, it is possible to deduce the absolute value of the dose received as well as the relative dose by measuring the relaxation rate R_2 ($R_2=1/T_2$) [146, 150].

Gel Dosimeter Characteristics. The requirements for an ideal dosimeters are as follows:

- high spatial resolution to be able to measure regions of steep dose gradient;
- three-dimensional (3-D) to be able to measure complex 3-D conformal dose distribution;
- dose integrating system to be able to deal with dynamically produced dose distributions;
- energy and dose rate independent to be able to give an absolute measure of the dose.

At the time of the experiment conducted in this work, gel dosimeters are believed to fulfil most of these criteria with the additional advantage of being tissue equivalent (density 0.99 $g.cm^{-1}$). Early results with the gel formulation used for the experiment have shown that the gel response is energy independent, see Table 6.5, and dose rate independent, see Table 6.6 (assuming an experimental error of 5%) [146, 150].

Table 6.5 Variation of relaxation rate $R_2=(1/T_2)$ with energy for an absorbed dose of 5 Gy

Energy	300 kV	Co-60 (4 MV)	6 MV	8 MV
Gel response R_2	1.68 ±0.08	1.69 ±0.08	1.76 ±0.08	1.68 ±0.08

Table 6.6 Variation of relaxation rate $R_2 = (1/T_2)$ with dose rate

Dose rate (Gy min^{-1})	1.6	2	2.8	4	5.5	8
Gel response R_2 (s^{-1})	4.08	4.19	4.22	4.1	4.23	4.3

It has also been shown that, as expected, the diffusion is not significant once that the gel has been irradiated. Similar to the film it is desirable to have a linear relationship between the gel response that is given by the relaxation rate R_2 and the absorbed dose. A typical calibration curve shown in Fig. 6.21 reveals that the response is linear up to 8-10 Gy.

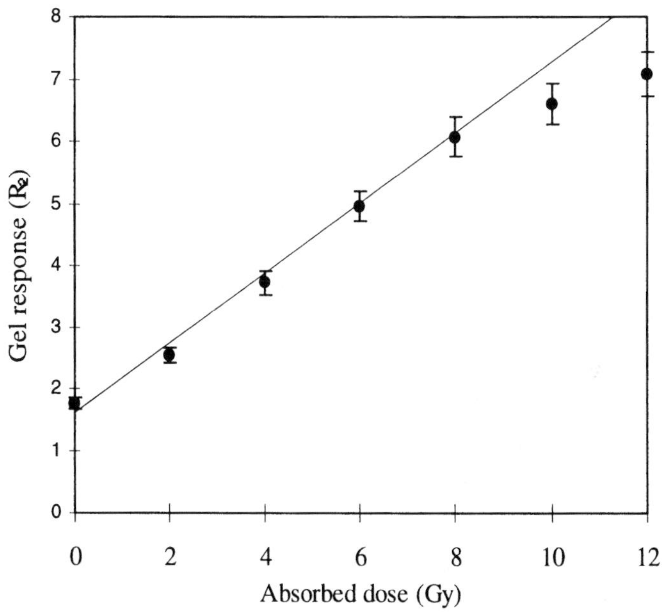

Fig. 6.21 Typical calibration curve for the gel manufactured at the Leicester Royal Infirmary

Experimental Set-up. The aim of this first experiment with BANG gel was both to assess the gel dosimeter and the ability of compensators to produce conformal treatments. It has been seen in the previous section that the gel can potentially give information on the absolute dose delivered as well as the relative dose. The first experiment carried out with used being made of film gave a global view of the distribution. This was particularly useful in assessing the relative dose distribution, especially the dose level close to the skin surface. In fact the film showed that no hot spots were present when use was made of the 25 MV beam. However it is believed that film did not provide the means to evaluate the dose distribution in the PTA area with sufficient accuracy. In order to overcome this problem use is made of gel dosimeter. Given the relatively high cost of the gel (£15 per litre, as opposed to £5 per film), and the limited quantity available at the time of the experiment, the gel was used solely to assess the dose distribution within a 10 cm diameter circle centred at the isocentre of the PTA. The experimental set up involved a more realistic phantom obtained from the cast of a patient treated at Walsgrave Hospital for prostate cancer. Whilst the shape of this torso phantom is similar, although smaller than the previous phantom used in conjunction with the film, the same compensators used for the first experiment were again utilised. Note that since the torso is smaller, different compensators would have been required to produce the same dose distribution as for the film. Making use of the same compensators, some beam weightings were slightly modified and a new dose distribution was predicted prior to subjecting the BANG gel dosimeter to the radiation field. The predicted dose distribution is given in Fig. 6.22.

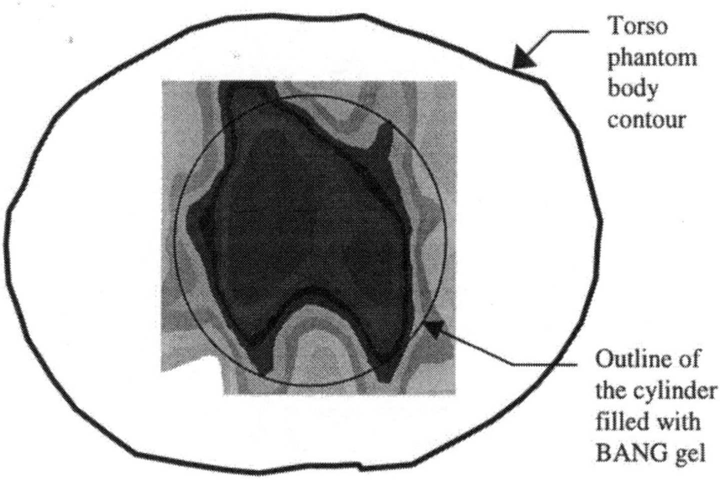

Fig. 6.22 Predicted dose distribution for more human like perspex torso phantom

The new torso phantom is hollow and can be viewed as a cylinder with one side opened, see Fig. 6.23. which shows the equipment used in the experiment involving the gel. A film holder or a smaller cylinder (10 cm in diameter) filled with gel dosimeter can be located in the middle of the torso phantom, and the phantom subsequently filled with water.

In order to accommodate for this open, cylinder like phantom, the procedure to administer the treatment had to be slightly modified. In the case of the slow film, the torso phantom was set up on the couch exactly as a patient would be, and the head of the linear accelerator was rotated around the patient. With this new torso phantom, it is required to position the phantom on the couch as if the patient were standing. This implies that in addition to the rotation of the head of the machine, it was necessary to rotate the couch. Depending on the position of the beam, the linac was rotated either by 90 degrees of 270 degrees so that it could be at right angles with the side of the phantom. The couch was then rotated by the required amount.

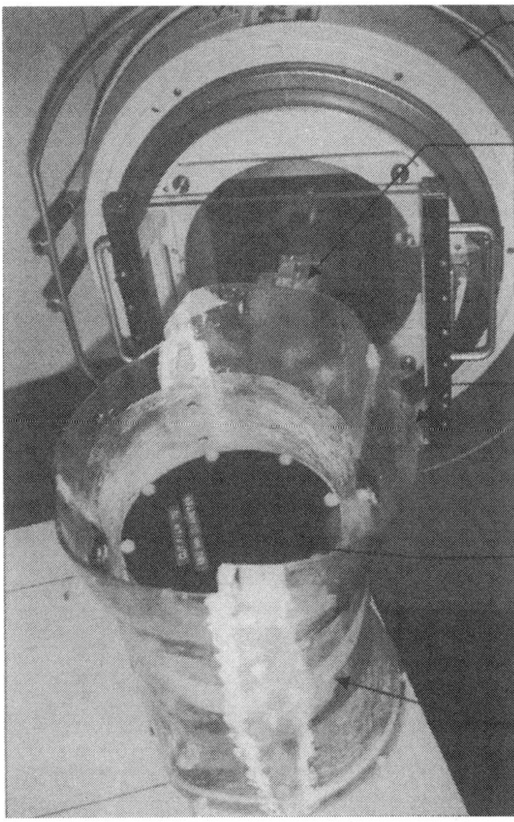

Fig. 6.23 Linear accelerator set up to assess a five field conformal dose distribution with film or gel dosimeter, courtesy of Walsgrave Hospital NHS Trust

After the experiment, the polymerisation in the gel was clearly visible. In fact even at this stage it could be observed that, at the location of the OAR within the PTA concavity, the gel was almost transparent, indicating that almost no polymerisation had occurred. This was later confirmed when the gel was imaged with an MRI scanner. The comparison between the distribution obtained from the processed output of the MRI scanner, represented by the shaded contour plot, and the densitometer for the film is illustrated in Fig. 6.24. In both cases, the relative dose distribution was normalised to 100%.

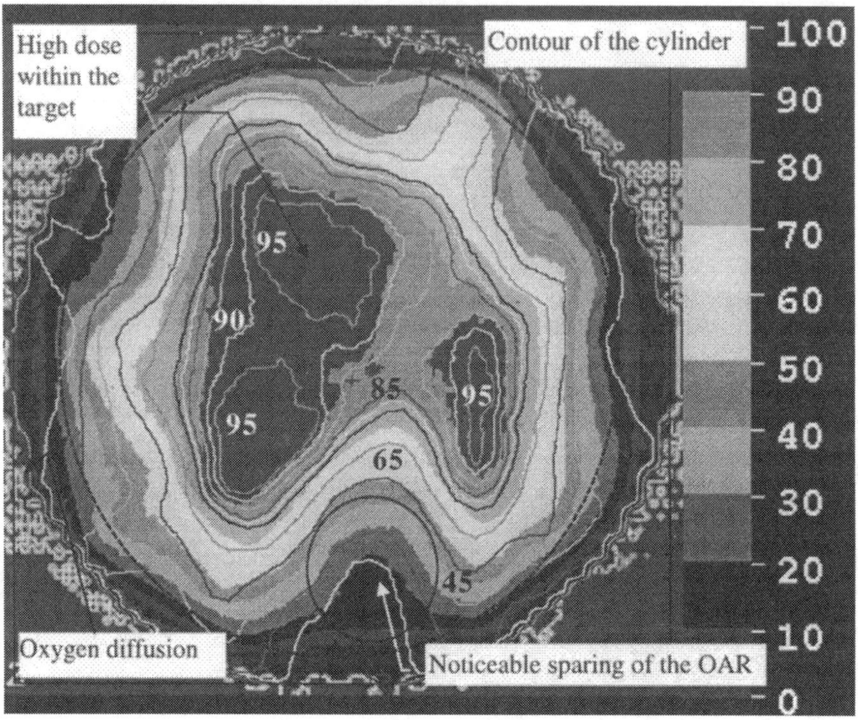

Fig. 6.24 Illustrating the comparison between dose distribution obtained from the film and the MRI scanner for the first practical demonstration of conformational radiotherapy using gel dosimeter in the UK

Overall results obtained with the BANG gel confirm earlier results obtained with the film. In particular, it can be observed that a very low dose is received by the OAR within the concavity of the PTA. Note that the fall-off of the dose on the edge of the circle is due to the lack of polymerisation process on the edge of the cylinder. This is due to the diffusion of oxygen through the perspex wall of the cylinder containing the gel. This oxygen diffusion has been found to affect the gel within 10 - 15 mm of the walls of the cylinder causing an underestimation of the dose. Such diffusion could have been prevented by the use of a glass cylinder and it is planned to repeat the experiment with such a container. In addition, at the time of the experiment, it was found that the gel could provide adequate relative dose distributions, with the absolute dose value being slightly overestimated. In particular, it appeared that the error in absolute dose value depended on the number of beams irradiating the gel. For the experiment 6 Gy were delivered and 7.5 ±0.5 Gy were measured. As a consequence only relative values have been considered in the work reported here.

6.4.3 Overall Assessment of the Experiment

The overall results of the experimental work conducted at Walsgrave Hospital NHS Trust have been considered to be very encouraging as they constituted the first attempt in the UK to actually realise beam intensity modulation [119, 147]. However, the actual realisation of intensity modulation via compensators was only made possible due to the preliminary modelling and dose distribution prediction as well as the actual realisation of the compensator devices themselves. In summary the experimental work has demonstrated that:

- The purpose developed parallel and divergent beam model can replicate adequately two-dimensional dose distributions of X-ray photon beams
- The beam orientation can be optimised on geometrical basis to conform to the PTA and spare OARs
- Conformal dose distributions can be predicted with the hybrid approach making use of ILS and MOGA (see Sect. 6.2)
- Compensator profiles can be calculated from IMB profiles produced by the hybrid optimisation algorithm
- Compensators can be manufactured relatively easily with a CNC machine to actually produce IMBs
- The shaping of the beams enables a noticeable sparing in the OARs to be achieved
- Conformal radiotherapy treatment plans can be delivered effectively with compensators

One of the most important factors in the actual delivery of the treatment was the accurate settings of the beams (i.e. field size, offset) and the positioning of the compensator on the tray. Indeed, even a beam offset as small as 0.5 cm could result in a very different dose distribution (recalling that organs may move by approximately 1 cm in the pelvic region). This confirms previous findings in [3, 4] which have shown that the actual importance of the positioning of all the elements of the linear accelerator with respect to the patient is further increased by the use of intensity modulated beams.

Inaccuracy can occur due to the measurement technique used. The film offers a relatively low resolution which may emphasise relatively small errors in the calculation of the number of monitor units to be delivered. In addition, the density of the torso phantom used with the film is considered to be identical to that of water, although it is slightly denser than water. Similarly, the gel used was slightly denser than water, however, this was not taken into account in the optimisation process.

One of the most important sources of error is believed to be the modelling of the compensator itself. Indeed the compensators were considered as two-dimensional devices whereas in fact they are inherently three-dimensional. Similarly the beam model used only accounts for two-dimensional scatter. The scaling up of the model from two-dimensions to three-dimensions is a clear area of further work.

6.5 Concluding Remarks

This Chapter has presented a practical verification of a global approach to the optimisation of X-ray photon beam intensity modulation for radiotherapy treatment. A hybrid approach that can potentially take into account the nature of the beam modulator has been used to adapt a theoretical solution found with ILS and a parallel beam model to a practicably implementable solution using a more realistic divergent beam model.

A relationship between the beam profiles and the compensator profiles has been proposed. The resulting compensator profile has then been altered to account for the diameter of the cutting tool prior creating a tool path to manufacture the compensator with a CNC machine. The results have been assessed using both well tried and novel experimental techniques. Radiosensitive film provides an overall view of the dose distribution, enabling the clinician to assess the dose distribution with respect to the relative dose level outside the PTA, whereas the BANG gel dosimeter enables a more precise assessment of the dose distribution within and around the PTA.

The results show that predicted and measured dose distributions are in good agreement. In particular, the conformal dose distributions obtained using this hybrid optimisation technique shows a significant sparing of the organs at risk that could not have been achieved using conventional techniques. The results are such that a full three-dimensional clinical application is now technically feasible.

CHAPTER 7
CONCLUSIONS

Unique to this monograph is the diversity yet interrelation of the radiotherapy treatment planning optimisation problems addressed. These range from the:

- optimisation of the number of beams and their respective orientation;
- optimisation of beam weights and wedge angles for standard radiotherapy;
- optimisation of the beam intensity modulation for intensity modulated radiation therapy.

By adopting a step by step approach each of these problems have been addressed and their solutions verified experimentally. The culmination of the work is a practical demonstration of intensity modulated radiation therapy, delivered via optimised patient specific compensators, under realistic clinical field trial conditions.

A key element to this approach was the use of systems modelling techniques to derive and evaluate a matrix based pencil beam model specifically designed to solve the so-called inverse problem in radiotherapy treatment planning; that is to work back from a clinical dose prescription to a set of intensity modulated beams. The developed model has been shown to satisfactorily replicate the characteristics of intensity modulated X-ray photon beams for 6 MV and 25 MV beam energies. The ability of the model to take into account the physical phenomenon of radiation scatter as well as the effect of inhomogeneities, penumbra, in-air-profile and irregularities in patient contours has also been demonstrated.

Software tools have been developed to optimise the number and orientation of beams prior to optimising the beam weights and wedge angles for traditional radiotherapy treatment or the beam in-field intensity modulation for intensity modulated radiation therapy.

Adopting a model based approach, the optimisation of beam intensity modulation is performed using a weighted iterative least squares (ILS) technique in a pseudo parallel manner. The approaches aim to determine an optimal solution in terms of minimising a least squares cost function which attempts to achieve a maximum uniform dose in the treatment area and minimum dose elsewhere; with particular emphasis being placed on the sparing of vital organs.

The initial ILS technique is modified to allow an adaptive scaling of the error to improve the performance of the general least squares algorithm. The influence of various modifications of the information matrix is studied and it is concluded that some of the schemes proposed are superior, both in terms of error and rate of convergence, to ILS with a fixed information matrix. The realisation of practical constraints, linked to the manufacture of compensators, has also been considered, with use being made of a cautious least squares scheme.

To overcome the recognised limitations of the ILS approaches, a procedure which could accommodate the potentially conflicting criteria that arises in the radiotherapy treatment planning problem was derived. In particular, multi-objective genetic algorithms (MOGAs) have been used to optimise intensity modulated beams, beam weight/wedge angle as well as coplanar beam orientation. The MOGAs developed exploit the concept of Pareto optimality which, when used together with progressive articulation of the objectives, can guide the search in an adaptive manner towards promising region of the solution space. Several 'decision makers' have also been developed to select a clinically appropriate solution from the Pareto optimal set determined by the MOGAs. A particular formulation was used to adapt the intensity modulated beam profiles, determined by making use of adaptive least squares in conjunction with a parallel beam model, to a more realistic fan beam model.

Another MOGA was hybridised to exploit a novel geometrical formulation of the objectives of radiotherapy treatment planning. A modified formulation of the objectives associated with the organs at risk was introduced to account for the different strategies that are required to be adopted when positioning the beams, for both traditional and more advanced intensity modulated radiotherapy techniques. An interesting observation was that not only will the approach give rise to the 'best' solution for a given number of beams, it can also give an indication of the minimum number of beams required in a given treatment plan.

Traditional beam compensation techniques making use of wedges have also been optimised using a hybrid MOGA. Of particular interest is the ability of the approach to produce well balanced treatment plans from within the solutions that are automatically included in the Pareto optimal set. This was found to overcome a common problem encountered by guided random search techniques used with a priori selection of the objectives, namely that of unbalanced plans with hot spots.

Finally all aspects of the work have been integrated and patient specific compensators have been manufactured and tested on a complex test case involving a five field treatment plan; this being representative of the type of treatment required in the pelvic region. A procedure for deducing the compensator profiles from the optimised intensity modulated beam profiles was presented. The approach developed is able to take into account tool path generation in the manufacture of the compensators.

All experimental work has been carried out at Walsgrave Hospital NHS Trust, Coventry, in the Department of Clinical Physics and Bioengineering. Measurements used to assess the effect of radiation from a single beam or from a combination of beams have been performed using two different linear accelerators.

A single energy linear accelerator was used in the experimental work involving a 6 MV photon beam, and a dual energy linear accelerator was used in the experimental work involving a higher energy 25 MV photon beam. The beam matrix based models developed were tuned using a water phantom positioned under the head of a linear accelerator.

Two different torso phantoms were used to assess the effect of intensity modulated beams produced by the patient specific compensators. A hardboard torso phantom was first used to assess the effect of intensity modulation both inside and outside the target region. A more realistic torso phantom was built in perspex from the cast of a cancer patient treated at Walsgrave Hospital NHS Trust, Coventry, to assess the dose distribution close to the target region. The latter was designed such that both film and gel dosimeter could be used to assess intensity modulated dose distributions. The manufacture and imaging of the experimental gel dosimeter was performed at Leicester Royal Infirmary, Leicester.

The outcomes of the experimental work show good agreement between the practical results obtained and the simulated theoretical predictions; thus reinforcing the validity and appropriateness of the overall approach. Indeed the results clearly show a sparing of the critical structures which could not have been achieved with conventional radiotherapy techniques.

The overall outcome of the work marks a significant milestone towards improving radiotherapy treatment and indicates clearly the potential of realising conformal radiotherapy using patient specific compensators. Results are very encouraging and the potential for reduced probability of complication and improved tumour controllability through accurate conformation and delivery of radiation makes the potential for improved quality of life after treatment a reality.

REFERENCES

[1] Haas OCL. Optimisation and control systems modelling in radiotherapy treatment planning. PhD thesis, Coventry University, UK, 1997

[2] Litcher AS, Ten Haken RK. Three-dimensional treatment planning and conformal radiation dose delivery. Important Advances in Oncology; 1995:95-105

[3] Smith AE (Ed). Radiotherapy Physics. Berlin Springer, Germany, 1995

[4] Webb S. The physics of three-dimensional radiation therapy: conformal therapy. radiosurgery and treatment planning. Institute of Physics Publishing, Bristol, 1993

[5] Brahme A. Optimisation of stationary and moving beam radiation therapy techniques. Radiotherapy and Oncology 1988; 12:129-140

[6] Mills JA, Jarvis R. Determination of beam profiles for conformation therapy using an iterative least squares technique. Institute of Physice in Science and Medecine/ British Institute of Radiology meeting, 1989

[7] Bortfeld T, Burkelbach J, Boesecke R and Schlegel W. Methods of image reconstruction from projections allpied to conformation therapy. Phys Med Biol 1990; 35(10):1423-1434

[8] Holmes T, Mackie RT. A filtered backprojection dose calculation for inverse treatment planning. Phys. Med. 1994; 21:303-313

[9] Hsia TC. System Identification. Lexington Books, 1977

[10] Reeves C R. Modern Heuristic Techniques for Combinatorial Problems. Blackwell Scientific Publications, 1993

[11] Fonseca C Multiobjective Genetic Algorithms with Application to Control Engineering Problems. PhD thesis, The University of Sheffield, UK, 1995

[12] Mould RF. A Century of Xrays and Radioactivity in Medicine. Institute of Physics Publishing. Bristol and Philadelphia, 1993

[13] Orton CG. Uses of therapeutic x rays in medicine. Health Physics 1995; 69(5):662-676

[14] Special Commemorative Issue 100 years of X-rays. Radiology Now 1995; 12

[15] 15th Annual European Society for Therapeutic Radiology and Oncology (ESTRO) Meeting. Vienna. Austria, Radiotherapy and Oncology 1996; 40(Suppl 1)

[16] Carol MP, Bleier AR, Campbell RC and Search JD. An automated 3-D conformal treatment planning system for linear accelerator based beam modulation

radiotherapy. Proc XIth Int Conf on the Use of Computers in Radiation Therapy (ICCR), Manchester, UK, 1994, pp 108-109

[17] Beavis AW, Weston SJ, Whitton VJ. Enhanced dynamic wedge - the comming of age of intensity modulated conformal therapy planning. Radiology UK 96, The British Journal of Radiology 1996; Suppl to vol. 69, p 99

[18] Dutching W, Ulmer W, Ginsberg T. Modelling of tumour growth and irradiaiton Proc XIth Int Conf on the Use of Computers in Radiation Therapy (ICCR), Manchester, UK 1994, pp 20-21

[19] Olsen DR. Calculation of the biological effect of fractionated radiotherapy: the importance of radiation-induced apoptosis. The British Journal of Radiology 1995; 68: 1230-1236

[20] Teo P ML, Kwan WH, Leung SF et al. Early tumour response and treatment toxicity after hyperfractionated radiotherapy in napharyngeal carcinoma. British Journal of Radiology 1996; 69:241-248

[21] Johnes B, Tan L T, Dale R G. Derivation of the optimum dose per fraction from the linear quadratic model. The British Journal of Radiology 1995; 68:894-902.

[22] Hirschfield F, Menke M, Rockel V, et al. Optical measurement and computer control of patient position and movement with newly developed system for fractionated radiotherapy. Proc XIth Int Conf on the Use of Computers in Radiation Therapy (ICCR), Manchester, UK, 1994, pp 108-9

[23] Hoskin PJ, Goodchild K, Powell M, Saunders MI. A phase I/II study of accelerated radiotherapy carbogen and nicotinamide in carcinoma of the bladder. Radiology UK 96, The British Journal of Radiology 1996; Suppl to vol. 69.

[24] Internal Commission on Radiolocal Units and Measurements. Prescribing. Recording and Reporting Photon Beam Therapy. ICRU Report 50 (ICRU, Bethesda, MD, USA). Washington DC, 1993

[25] Central Axis Depth Dose for Use in Radiotherapy. The British Journal of Radiology 1983; Suppl 17

[26] Central Axis Depth Dose for Use in Radiotherapy. The British Journal of Radiology; 1996; Suppl 25

[27] Bortfeld T, Schlegel W. Optimisation of beam orientation in radiation therapy: some theoretical considerations. Phys Med. Biol; 1993; 38:291-304

[28] Haas OCL, Burnham KJ, Mills JA. Optimization of beam orientation in radiotherapy using planar geometry, Phys Med Biol 1998;43:2179-2193

[29] Gokhale P, Hussein MA, Kulkarni N. Determination of beam orientation in radiotherapy planning. Med Phys 1994; 21(3):393-400.

[30] Ezzell GA. Genetic and geometric optimization of three-dimensional radiation therapy treatment planning Med Phys 1996; 23(3):293-305

[31] Yu CX, Yan D, Du MN, Zhou S, Verhey LJ. Optimization of leaf positions when shaping a radiation field with a multileaf collimator. Phys Med Biol 1995; 40:305-308.

[32] Fernandez EM, Shentall GS, Mayles WPM, Dearnaley DP. The acceptability of a multileaf collimator as a replacement for conventional blocks. Radiotherapy and Oncology 1995; 36:65-74

[33] Horwich A, Wynne C, Nahum A, Swindell W, Dearnaley DP. Conformal radiotherapy at the Royal Marsden Hospital. Int J Radiat Biol 1994; 65(1):117-122

[34] Hounsel AR, Marrs JE, Moore CJ, Sharrock PJ, Shaw AJ, Wilkinson JM. High technology to simplify the planning and delivery of radiotherapy, Radiotherapy and Oncology 1993; 29:192-196

[35] Moore C. Computerised conformal radiation therapy - a critical process. IEE. Computing & Control Engineering Journal 1995, Oct

[36] Oldham M, Webb S. Inverse planning and the optimisation of radiotherapy plans by simulated annealing incorporating dual weighting. Proc. XIth Int. Conf. on the Use of Computers in Radiation Therapy(ICCR), Manchester, UK, 1994, pp 60-61

[37] Oldham M, Webb S. The optimization and inherent limitations of 3D conformal radiotherapy treatment plans of the rostate. The British Journal of Radiology 1995; 68: 882-893

[38] Wilks R, Casebow MP. Tissue compensation with lead for ^{60}Co therapy. The British Journal of Radiology 1969; 42: 452-456

[39] Renner WD, O'Connor TP, Bermudez NM. An algorithm for design of beam compensators. Int J Radiation Oncology Biol Phys 1989; 17: 227-234

[40] Djordjevich A. Bonham DJ. Hussien EMA. Andrew JW. Hale ME. Optimal design of radiation compensators. Med Phys 1990; 17:397-404

[41] Mageras GS, Mohan R, Burman C, Barest GD, Kutcher GJ. Compensators for three-dimensional treatment planning. Med Phys 1991; 18:133-140

[42] Jursinic PA, Podgorsak B, Paliwal BR. Implementation of a three-dimensional compensating system based on computed tomography generated surface contours and tissue inhomogeneities. Med Phys 1994; 21:357-365

[43] Li C. photon beam compensation design: dose optimisation in 3D volume for parallel opposed beams. Medical Dosimetry 1993; 18:197-202

[44] Kallman P, Lind B, Ecklof A, Brahme A. Shaping of arbitrary dose distributions by dynamic multi-leaf collomation. Phys Med Biol 1988; 11:1291-1300

[45] Bortfeld T, Kahler D, Waldron T, Boyer A. X-ray field compensation with multileaf collimators. Int J Radiation Oncology Biol Phys; 1994; 28 (3), : 723-730

[46] Svenson R, Kallman P, Brahme A. Realisation of physical and biological dose optimisation using dynamic multileaf collimation. Proc XIth Int Conf on the Use of Computers in Radiation Therapy (ICCR), Manchester, UK, 1994, pp 56-57

[47] Svenson R, Kallman P, Brahme A. An analytical solution for the dynamic control multileaf collimators. Phys Med Biol 1994; 39:37-61

[48] Aoki Y, Nakagawa K, Onogi Y, Sasaki Y, Akanuma A. Coplanar verses non coplanar dose optimisation with multileaf collimator. Proc XIth Int Conf on the Use of Computers in Radiation Therapy (ICCR), Manchester, UK, 1994, pp 12-13

[49] Boyer AL, Bortfeld T, Schlegel W, Kahler DL, Waldron TJ. MLC modulation of X-ray beams in discrete steps. Proc XIth Int Conf on the Use of Computers in Radiation Therapy (ICCR). Manchester, UK, 1994, pp 178-79

[50] Bortfeld T, Boyer AL, Schlegel W, Kahler DL, Waldron TJ. Experimental verification of modulated conformal radiotherapy. Proc XIth Int Conf on the Use of Computers in Radiation Therapy (ICCR). Manchester, UK, 1994, pp 180-81

[51] Innes GS. The one million volt X-ray therapy equipment at St Bartholomew's Hospital. 1936-1960. Proc Megavoltage Radiotherapy 1937-1987, British Journal of Radiology 1988; Suppl to vol. 22

[52] Johnes AE. The development of megavoltage X-ray therapy at St Bartholomew's Hospital. Proc Megavoltage Radiotherapy 1937-1987, British Journal of Radiology 1988; Suppl to vol. 22

[53] Attix FH. Introduction to radiological physics and radiation dosimetry. John Wiley & Sons, 1986

[54] Fabrikant JI, Levy RP, Steinberg MD, Phillips MH, Frankel KA, Lynman JT, Marks MP, Silverberg GD. Charged particle radiosurgery for intracranial vascular malformations. Stereotactic radiosurgery 1992; 3(1) 99-139

[55] Chauvel P. Treatment planning with heavy ions. Radiat Environ Biophys 1995; 34: 49-53

[56] Coquard R, Ginestet C, Sentenac I, Carrie C, Gerard JP. La radiothérapie de conformation en 1995: acquis technologiques et perspectives cliniques. Bull Cancer/Radiother 1995; 82: 40-50

[57] Bueno MG. Computer aided segmentation of anatomical structures in computed tomographic images. PhD thesis, Coventry University, UK, 1998

[58] Pross J, Bendl R, Schlegel W. TOMAS. a tool for manual segmentation based on multiple image data sets. Proc XIth Int Conf on the Use of Computers in Radiation Therapy (ICCR), Manchester, UK, 1994, pp 192-3

[59] Cunningham JR. Scatter-air ratios. Phys Med Biol 1972, 17:42-51

[60] Tait DM, Nahum AE. Conformal therapy. Eur J Cancer 1990, 26(6):750-753

[61] Raphael C. Mathematical modelling of objectives in radiation therapy treatment planning. Phys Med Biol 1992; 37:1293-1311

[62] Ford J. Computer revolution in radiation therapy. Proc XIth Int Conf on the Use of Computers in Radiation Therapy (ICCR). Manchester. UK. March. pp 208-9. 1994

[63] Rosenman J. Future directions in 3-Dimensional Radiation Treatment planning. Oncology 1993; 7:11

[64] The British Standard Institution (BSI) 5724 section 31. ISE 976 1989. Medical Electrical Equipment Methods of Declaring Functional Performence Characteristics of Medical Electronic Accelerator in the Range 1 MeV 50 MeV, 1990

[65] Gray K, Smith CW. Accuracy of dose calculation methods for retracted tissue compensators. Phys Med Biol 1994; 39:2355-2365

[66] El-Khatib EE, Podgorsak EB, Pla C. The effect of lead attenuators on dose on homogeneous phantoms. Med Phys 1986; 13:928-935

[67] Touboul E, Lefkopoulos D. Radiotherapie de conformation tridimensionnelle: Compte rendu du 3D radiation treatment planning and conformal therapy An international symposium 21 au 23 avril 1993 à Saint-Louis. Missouri. Etats-Unis. Bull Cancer/ Radiother 1994; 81:7-21

[68] Brahme A, Lind B, Kallman P. Inverse radiation therapy planning as a tool for 3D dose optimisation. Physics Medica 1990; 6:53-68

[69] Brahme A. Inverse radiation therapy planning: principles and possibilities. Proc XIth Int Conf on the Use of Computers in Radiation Therapy (ICCR). Manchester. UK. March. 1994, pp 6-7.

[70] Stein J. Bortfeld T. Dorschel B. Schlegel W. X-ray intensity modulation by dynamic multileaf collimation. Proc XIth Int Conf on the Use of Computers in Radiation Therapy (ICCR). Manchester, UK, 1994, pp 174-75

[71] Wang X, Spirou S, LoSasso T, Stein J, Chui SC, Mohan R. Dosimetric verification of intensity-modulated fields, Med. Phys. 1996; 23(3):317-327

[72] Holmes T Mackie RT. A comparison of three inverse treatment planning algorithms. Phys Med Biol 1994; 39: 91-106

[73] Mackie TR. Holmes T. Reckwerdt P. Deasy OJ. Yang J. Paliwal B. Kinsella T. Tomotherapy: a new concept for the delivery of dynamic conformal radiotherapy. Med Phys 1993; 20 (6) pp 1709-1719

[74] Holmes TW. Mackie RT. Reckwerdt P. Deasy OJ. A prototype inverse treatment planning algorithm for tomotherapy. Proc XIth Int Conf on the Use of Computers in Radiation Therapy (ICCR). Manchester, UK, 1994, pp 62-3.

[75] Mackie TR. Holmes T. Reckwerdt P. Yang J. Swerdloff S. Deasy OJ. DELuca PM. Paliwal B. Kinsella T. Tomotherapy: a proposal for dedicated computer controlled delivery and verification system for conformational radiotherapy. Proc XIth Int Conf on the Use of Computers in Radiation Therapy (ICCR). Manchester, UK, 1994, pp 176-78.

[76] Carol MP. Integrated 3-D conformal multivane intensity modulation delivery system for radiotherapy. Proc XIth Int Conf on the Use of Computers in Radiation Therapy (ICCR). Manchester, UK, 1994, pp 172-73

[77] Carol MP et al. The matchline problem as it applies to the peackock 3-D conformal system. 35th ASTRO meeting. Rad Oncol Biol Phys 1995; 27(1):209

[78] Woo SY. Grant III WH. Bellezza D. Grossman R. Gildenberg P. Carpenter LS. Carol M. Butler EB. A comparison of intensity modulated conformal therapy with a conventional external beam stereotactic radiosurgery system for the treatment of single and multiple intracranial lesions. Int J Radiation Oncology Biol Phys 1996; 35(3):593-597

[79] Fallowfield L The Quality of Life. The Missing Measurement in Health Care. Human Horizons Series. Souvenir Press. 1990

[80] Söderström S. Gustafsson A. Brahme A. The clinical value of different treatment objectives and degree of freedom in radiation therapy optimization. Radiotherapy and Oncology 1993; 29:148-163.

[81] Nimierko A. Goitein M. Implementation of a model for estimating tumor control probability for an inhomogeneously irradiated tumour. Radiotherapy and Oncology 1993; 29:140-147

[82] Webb S. Nahum AE. A model for calculating tumour control probability in radiotherapy including the effects of inhomogeneous dirtributions of dose and clonogenic cell density. Phys Med Biol 1993; 38:653-666.

[83] Bortfeld T, Stein J, Preiser K. Clinically relevant intensity modulation optimisation using physical criteria, Proc. of the 12th Int. Conf. on the use of Computers in Radiation Therapy, Salt Lake City, UT, (eds) D.D. Leavitt and G. Starkschall, 1997, (Medical Physics, Madison, WI) pp 1-4

[84] Redpath AT. Vickery BL Wright DH. A new technique for radiotherapy planning using quadratic programming. Phys Med Biol 1976; 21: 781-791

[85] Steuer RE. Multiple criteria optimization: Theory. Computation. and Application. Wiley & Sons, 1986

[86] Petti PL. Siddon RL. Effective wedge angles with a universal wedge. Phys Med Biol 1985; 9: 985-991

[87] Mageras GS. Mohan R. Application of fast simulated annealing to optimization of conformal radiation treatments. Med Phys, 1993; 20(3): 639-647

[88] Morill S. Lane R. Jacobson G. Rosen I. Treatment planning optimisation using constrained simulated annealing. Phys Med Biol 1991; 36(10): 1341-1361

[89] Nimierko A. Random search algorithm (RONSC) for optimization of radiation therapy with both physical and Biological end points and constraints. Int J Radiation Oncology Biol Phys 1992; 23:89-98

[90] Nimierko A. Urie M. Goitein M. Optimisation of 3D radiation therapy with both physical and Biological end points and constraints. J Radiation Oncology Biol Phys 1992; 23:99-108

[91] Mageras GS. Podmanicky KC. Mohan R. A model for computer controlled delivery of 3-D conformal treatments. Med Phys 1992; 19(4):945-953

[92] Langer M. Brown R. Morrill S. Lane R. Lee O. A generic genetic algorithm for generating beam intensities. AAPM. Med Phys: 1994, 878

[93] Censor Y.Altschuler MD. Powlis D. On the use of Cimmino's simultaneous projections method for computing a solution of the inverse problem in radiation therapy treatment planning. Inverse Problems 1988; 4:607-623

[94] Censor YA. .Altschuler MD. Powlis D. computational solution of the inverse problem in radiation treatment planning. Applied Mathematics and Computation 1988; 25:57-87

[95] McShan DL. Conformal treatment planning. AMPI Medical Physics Bulletin 1990; 15.(3&4):190-199

[96] Webb S. Optimisation by Simulated Annealing of three-dimensional. conformal treatment planning for radiation fields defined by a multileaf collimator. Phys Med Biol 1991; 36(9):1201-1226

[97] Webb S. Optimisation by Simulated Annealing of three-dimensional. conformal treatment planning for radiation fields defined by a multileaf collimator: II Inclusion of two -dimensional modulation of the x-ray intensity. Phys Med Biol 1991; 36(9):1689-1704

[98] Gustafsson A. Lind BK. Brahme A. A generalized algorithm for optimization of radiation therapy. Proc XIth Int Conf on the Use of Computers in Radiation Therapy (ICCR). Manchester, UK, 1994, pp 68-9

[99] Holmes T. Mackie RT. Simpkin D. Reckwerdt P. A unified approach to the optimisation of brachytherapy and external beam dosimetry. Int J Radiation Oncology Biol Phys 1991;20:859-873

[100] Yuan Y. Sandham WA. Durrani TS. Mills JA. Deehan C. Application of Bayesian and maximum entropy to conformation radiotherapy treatment planning. Applied Sig Process 1994; 20(1):20-34

[101] Lind BK. Properties of an algorithm for solving the inverse problem. Inverse problem 1990; 6:415-426

[102] Holmes T. A model for the Physical Optimization of External Beam Radiotherapy. PhD thesis. University of Wisconsin-Madison. USA. 1993

[103] Yuan Y. Sandham WA. Durrani TS. Towards beam based optimisation for conformation RTP. Proc XIth Int Conf on the Use of Computers in Radiation Therapy (ICCR). Manchester, UK, 1994, pp 250-1

[104] Haas OCL, Burnham KJ, Fisher MH, Mills J.A, Genetic algorithm applied to radiotherapy treatment planning, Proc. Int. Conf. Artificial Neural Networks and Genetic Algorithms ICANNGA 95, Ales, Fr, 1995, pp 432-435

[105] Bartec TPS V. Physics manual. Chapter 1. external beam planning - photons. 1990

[106] Haas OCL, Burnham KJ, Fisher MH, Mills JA, Development of optimisation algorithms for conformation therapy, Radiology & Oncology 94, British Journal of Radiology, Harrogate, UK, 1994 Suppl. to vol. 67, Work in Progress

[107] Haas OCL, Burnham KJ, Mills JA, Formulation of beam profile determination problem for conformation therapy, Proc. Int. AMSE Conference "Systems", vol. 4 London, UK, Sept. 1-3, AMSE Press, 1993, pp 191-200

[108] Haas OCL, Burnham KJ, Fisher MH, Mills JA, A comparison of optimisation techniques for use in conformation therapy, Proc. Int. Conf. System Engineering, ICSE94, vol.. 1, Coventry, UK, Coventry University,1994, pp 434-442

[109] Mohan R. Chui CS. Lidofsky L. Differential pencil beam dose computation model for photons. Med Phys 1986; 13:64-73

[110] Mohan R. Chui CS. Validity of the concept of separating primary and scatter dose. Med Phys 1985; 12:726-731

[111] Redpath AT. Aspratakis MM. A beam model for three-dimensional photon treatment planning. Proc XIth Int Conf on the Use of Computers in Radiation Therapy (ICCR). Manchester, UK, 1994, pp 236-237

[112] Haas. OCL. Beam Profile Determination for Conformation Therapy. MSc Dissertation. Coventry University. September 1993

[113] Matlab. Matrix manipulation software. 1993

[114] Wood RG. Computer In Radiotherapy - Physical aspects. Computer in Medecine Series. Butterworth & Co. 1974

[115] Ahnesjö A. Saxner M. TreppA. A pencil beam model for photon dose calculation. Med Phys 1992; 19(2):263-274

[116] Cassell KJ. Hobday A. Parker RP. The implementation of a generalised Batho inhomogeneity correction for radiotherapy planning with direct use of CT numbers. Phys Med Biol 1981; 26

[117] Gover MJC. Barnett S. Properties of Toeplitz and Toeplitz-like matrices. and solutions of systems of linear equations with patterned coefficient matrices. Proc V Polish-English Seminar on Real-Time Process Control. Radziejowice, Poland, 1986 pp 150-159.

[118] Haas OCL, Burnham KJ, Mills JA. Improving physical selectivity in the treatment of cancer: a systems modelling and optimisation approach. International Federation of Automatic Control (IFAC) Biomedical Symposium, Warwick, UK, 1997

[119] Haas OCL, Burnham KJ, Mills JA. On improving physical selectivity in the treatment of cancer: a systems modelling and optimisation approach. Control Engineering Practice 1997; 12(5):1739-1745

[120] Vance R, Sandham W, Durrani T. Optimisation of beam profiles in conformational therapy using genetic algorithms. 35th American Soceity for Therapeutic Radiology and Oncology ASTRO meeting, pp 518, 1994

[121] Fletcher R. Practical Methods of Optimization. Volume 1 Unconstrained Optimisation. John Wiley & Sons. 1980

[122] Fletcher R. Practical Methods of Optimization. Volume 2 Constrained optimisation. John Wiley & Sons. 1981

[123] Burnham KJ. Self Tuning Control for Bilinear Systems. PhD thesis, Coventry Polytechnic, UK 1991

[124] Young PC. Recursive approach to time series analysis. Bulletin of IMA 1974; 10:209-224

[125] Strang G Linear Algebra and its Applications. Academic Press. London. UK. 2nd Ed. 1980

[126] Haas OCL, Burnham KJ, Fisher MH, Mills JA. Use of genetic algorithms in radiotherapy treatment planning,. Neural Networks and Expert Systems in Medicine and Healthcare (NNESMED'96), Plymouth, UK, 1996, pp 275-283

[127] Haas OCL, Burnham KJ, Fisher MH, Mills JA, Beam Orientation and intensity modulation for conformation therapy, 15th Annual European Society of Therapeutic Radiology and Oncology (ESTRO) Meeting, Radiotherapy & Oncology, Vienna, Austria, 1996 (40 Suppl. 1):182

[128] Haas OCL, Burnham KJ, Fisher MH, Mills JA, Implementation of hot spot correction schemes for use in optimisation algorithms for conformation therapy, Radiology UK 96, Birmingham, UK, British Journal of Radiology, 1996, (Suppl. to vol. 69):100

[129] Deasy JO. De Leone R. Holmes TW. Mackie TR. Beam weight optimisation using the MIMOS computer code. Proc XIth Int Conf on the Use of Computers in Radiation Therapy (ICCR). Manchester, UK, 1994, pp 64-5.

[130] Haas OCL, Burnham KJ, Mills JA, Adaptive error weighting scheme to solve the inverse problem in radiotherapy, Proc. 12th Int. Conf. on Systems Engineering, ICSE'97, Coventry University, UK, 1997, pp 290-295

[131] Goldberg DE. Genetic algorithms in Search Optimization & Machine Learning. Addison-Wesley. 1989

[132] Alander JA. An Indexed Bibliography of Genetic Algorithm in Control. ftpuwasafi. /cs/report94-1. gaCONTROLbibpsZ. 1995

[133] Beightler CS. Phillips DT. Wilde DJ. Foundations of Optimization 2nd Ed.Prentice-Hall. 1979

[134] Daellenbach HD. George JA. Introduction to Operations Research Techniques. Allyn and Bacon. 1978

[135] Metropolis N, Rosenbluth AW, Rosenbluth MN, Teller AH, Teller E. Equation of state calculation by fast computing machines. J of Chem Phys 1953; 21:1087-1091

[136] Kirkpatrick S, Gellat CD, Vecchi MP. Optimisation by simulated annealing. Science 1983; 220:671-680

[137] Otten RHJM, Ginneken LPPP. The annealing algorithm. Kluwer academic publisher. 1989

[138] Hwang CL, Masud ASM. Multiple Objective Decision Making - Methods and Applications. volume 164 of Lecture Notes in Economics and Mathematical Systems. Springer-Verlag. Berlin. 1979

[139] Haas OCL, Burnham KJ, Fisher MH, Mills JA, Genetic algorithms applied to beam orientation in radiotherapy, Proc. Fourth European Congress an Intelligent Techniques and Soft Computing (EUFIT 96), vol. 3, Aachen, Germany, 1996; pp 2050-2055

[140] Stein J, Mohan R, Wang X-H, Bortfeld T, Wu Q, Ling C C and Schelgel W. Number and orientation of beams in intensity-modulated radiation treatments. Med. Phys. 1997; 24(2):149-160

[141] Söderström S and Brahme A. Which is the most suitable number of photon beam portal in coplanar radiation therapy. Int. J. Radiation Oncology Biol. Phys. 1995; 33(1):151-159

[142] Chipperfield. Fleming. Polheim. Fonseca. Genetic Algorithm toobox for MATLAB. 1995

[143] Phillips Medical System Division 1983. Product Data 764 (Eindoven: Philips)

[144] Sherouse G.W., A mathematical basis for selection of wedge angle and orientation, *Med. Phys.*, **20** (4), 1993

[145] Mining Chemical Product. safety data sheet No 56. issue 2. 1996

[146] Haas OCL, Mills JA, Burnham KJ, Bonnet DE, Farajollani AR, Fisher MH, Glendinning AG and Aukett RJ, Experimental verification of beam intensity modulated conformal radiotherapy using patient specific compensators, Radiology 1997, Imaging, Science & Oncology, Birmingham, UK, British Journal of Radiology, 1997, (Suppl. to vol. 70):16-17

[147] Haas OCL, Mills JA, Burnham KJ, Bonnett DE, Farajollahi AR, Achieving conformal dose distribution via patient specific compensators, XII Int. Conf. on the use of computers in radiation therapy, XII ICCR, Salt Lake City, USA, 1997, p 483

[148] Fricke H. Hart EJ. Radiation Dosimetry. vol 2. Ed FH Attix and WC Roesch (New York: Academic), 1966

[149] Maryanski MJ. Schulz RJ. Ibbott GS. Gatenby JC. Xie J. Horton D and Gore JC. Magnetic resonance imaging of radiation dose distributions using polymer-gel dosimeter. Phys Med Biol 1994; 39:1437-1455.

[150] Bonnet DE, Farajollani AR, Haas OCL, Mills JA, Glendinning AG, Aukett RJ, Burnham K., The verification of intensity modulated conformal therapy using polymer gel dosimetry, Specialised Treatment Techniques, Dosimetry and Verification Meeting organised by the Institution of Physics & Engineering in Medecine & Biology (IPEMB), London, UK, 1997

INDEX

Made in the USA
Monee, IL
13 September 2026

62976975R00136